MW01034288

Clinical Pocket Guide to Advanced Practice Palliative Nursing

Clinical Pocket Guide to Advanced Practice Palliative Nursing

Edited by

Constance Dahlin, MSN, ANP-BC, ACHPN, FPCN, FAAN

Director of Professional Practice
Hospice and Palliative Nurses Association
Pittsburgh, Pennsylvania
Palliative Nurse Practitioner
North Shore Medical Center
Salem, Massachusetts

Patrick J. Coyne, MSN, ACNS-BC, ACHPN, FAAN, FPCN

Director of Palliative Care
Medical University of South Carolina
Charleston, South Carolina

Betty R. Ferrell, PhD, RN, MA, CHPN, FAAN, FPCN

Professor and Director of Nursing Research and Education
City of Hope Comprehensive Cancer Center
Duarte, California

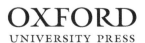

OXFORD
UNIVERSITY PRESS

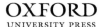

OXFORD
UNIVERSITY PRESS

Oxford University Press is a department of the University of Oxford. It furthers
the University's objective of excellence in research, scholarship, and education
by publishing worldwide. Oxford is a registered trade mark of Oxford University
Press in the UK and certain other countries.

Published in the United States of America by Oxford University Press
198 Madison Avenue, New York, NY 10016, United States of America.

© Oxford University Press 2017

Library of Congress Cataloging-in-Publication Data
Names: Dahlin, Constance, editor. | Coyne, Patrick, 1957- editor. | Ferrell, Betty, editor.
Title: The clinical pocket guide to advanced practice palliative nursing /
edited by Constance Dahlin, Patrick J. Coyne, Betty Ferrell.
Description: Oxford ; New York : Oxford University Press, [2017] |
Includes bibliographical references.
Identifiers: LCCN 2016042545 | ISBN 9780190204709 (pbk. : alk. paper)
Subjects: | MESH: Hospice and Palliative Care Nursing--methods |
Advanced Practice Nursing—methods | Handbooks
Classification: LCC RT87.T45 | NLM WY 49 | DDC 616.02/9—dc23
LC record available at https://lccn.loc.gov/2016042545

Contents

Preface

Advancing Palliative Nursing

We offer this handbook to the bedside advanced practice registered nurse (APRN) who is dedicated to quality palliative nursing. We know it takes courage, strength, skills, knowledge, and energy to do this, given the ever-changing sands of healthcare.

This handbook is created from the *Advanced Practice Palliative Nursing* textbook. In order to create this handbook, we took key chapters from the textbook that focused on clinical care. It is our intention to provide a quick reference for the clinical APRN. There are thousands of specialty APRNs providing palliative care within oncology, cardiology, and neurology, to name just a few. While some people have felt there were bedside palliative medicine quick reference guides, we wanted to assure a quick handbook that reflected advanced practice palliative nursing and provided consistency in the nursing process from assessment to management and evaluation of pain, symptoms, and various situations.

We appreciate our authors' contributions to this project. We understand that the time they devoted to this project took away from their own personal time, family time, or "down time."

These topics were determined based on our previous experience in educating our colleagues. The authors are practicing clinicians who understand the practice of palliative care and can speak to the issues of care delivery. The book is grounded in the domains of the National Consensus Project for Quality Palliative Care's *Clinical Practice Guidelines for Quality Palliative Care*, as well as the standards and competencies of the American Nurses Association and the Hospice and Palliative Nurses Association's *Palliative Nursing: Scope and Standards—An Essential Resource*.

Audience

This text is intended for graduate nursing students, practicing palliative APRNs, and graduate-prepared advanced practice nurses interested in palliative care but who work in nonclinical settings such as research, academia, and administration. We think this text will provide a comprehensive resource to consider clinical issues and future directions for palliative APRN policy.

We also hope it promotes role development within the spectrum of APRN practice. For practicing APRNs, the book promotes skills and competencies as a foundation for advanced practice palliative nursing practice. For educators, the book offers a curricular resource in preparing the next generation of palliative APRNs.

Contributors

Vanessa Battista, MSN, RN, CPNP
Pediatric Advanced Care Team
The Children's Hospital of
    Philadelphia
Philadelphia, Pennsylvania

Ann Berger, MSN, MD
Chief of Pain and Palliative Care
National Institutes of Health
    Clinical Center
Bethesda, Maryland

Barton T. Bobb, MSN, FNP-BC, ACHPN
Virginia Commonwealth University
    Health System
Massey's Thomas Palliative
    Care Services
Richmond, Virginia

Kathleen Broglio, DNP, ANP-BC, ACHPN
Senior Nurse Practitioner
Adult Ambulatory Palliative
    Care Services
Columbia University Medical Center
New York, New York

Marcia J. Buckley MSN, OCNS, ANP, ACHPN
Senior Nurse Practitioner
Palliative Care Consultation Service
University of Rochester Medical
    Center, Strong Hospital
Associate Professor of Clinical
    Nursing
University of Rochester School
    of Nursing
Adjunct Faculty
St. John Fisher College
Rochester, New York

Peggy S. Burhenn, MS, CNS, AOCNS
Professional Practice Leader
City of Hope Comprehensive
    Cancer Center
Duarte, California

John D. Chovan, PhD, DNP, CNP, CNS, PMHNP-BC, ACHPN, AHN-BC
Assistant Professor and Director,
    DNP Program
Department of Nursing
Otterbein University
Westerville, Ohio
Nurse Practitioner
Mount Carmel Hospice and
    Palliative Care
Columbus, Ohio

Kimberly Chow, MSN, ANP-BC, ACHPN
Memorial Sloan-Kettering
    Cancer Center
New York, New York

Devon Fletcher, MD
Virginia Commonwealth University
    Health System
Massey's Thomas Palliative Care
    Services
Richmond, Virginia

Maria Gatto, MA, NP, HNP, APRN-BC, ACHPN
Trinity Health System Director,
    Palliative Care
Trinity Health
Livonia, Michigan

Janine A. Gerringer, MSN, CRNP
Ventricular Assist Device
    Coordinator
Geisinger Health System
Danville, Pennsylvania

Lauren Koranteng, PharmD, CPE
Memorial Sloan-Kettering
    Cancer Center
New York, New York

Maureen Lynch, MS, ANP-BC, AOCN, ACHPN, FPCN
Nurse Practitioner
Division of Palliative Care
Dana Farber Cancer Institute
Boston, Massachusetts

Patricia Maani Fogelman, DNP
Director of Thoracic Medicine
GMC Nursing Grand Rounds
Associate Professor of Nursing
Columbia University
New York, New York

Peg Nelson, MSN, NP, ACHPN
Director of Palliative Care and Pain
    Services
St. Joseph Mercy Oakland
Pontiac, Michigan

Judith A. Paice, PhD, RN, FAAN
Director of the Cancer Pain
    Program
Division of Hematology-Oncology
Northwestern University
Feinberg School of Medicine
Chicago, Illinois

Kathy Plakovic, MSN, FNP-BC, ACHPN
Palliative Care Nurse Practitioner
Edward Hospital
Naperville, Illinois

Gina Santucci, MSN, APRN-BC
Pediatric Advanced Care Team
The Children's Hospital of
    Philadelphia
Philadelphia, Pennsylvania

Ann Syrett, MS, FNP-BC, ACHPN
Nurse Practitioner
Palliative Care Consultation Service
University of Rochester Medical
    Center, Strong Hospital
Rochester, New York

Patricia Thomas, PhD, RN
Vice President Clinical Quality &
    Transformation/Chief Nursing
    Officer
Trinity Home Health Services
Livonia, Michigan

Beth Wagner, MSN, CRNP, ACHPN
Nurse Practitioner
Palliative Care Team
Thomas Jefferson University
    Hospital
Philadelphia, Pennsylvania

Phyllis B. Whitehead, PhD, APRN, RN-BC, ACHPN
Clinical Nurse Specialist
Palliative Care Service at Carilion
    Roanoke Memorial Hospital
Assistant Professor
Virginia Tech Carilion School of
    Medicine
Roanoke, Virginia

Clinical Pocket Guide to Advanced Practice Palliative Nursing

Chapter 1

Pain

Judith A. Paice

Key Points

- Expert assessment skills are essential to effective pain management in palliative care.
- Comprehensive knowledge of pain management options includes appropriate therapies, safe and effective medication use, and essential interventions, such as physical or occupational therapy, interventional techniques, and cognitive-behavioral strategies.
- Safe prescribing practices are vital for patients, families, and society at large.

Pain Syndromes in Palliative Care

Differentiating acute from chronic pain syndromes will help determine the course and treatment options (Box 1.1).[1]

Another strategy for grouping pain syndromes is by their quality: somatic, neuropathic, visceral, or mixed.[5]

- Somatic pain—usually managed by nonopioids and opioids
- Neuropathic pain—treated with adjuvant analgesics and opioids (little or no response to nonopioids)
- Visceral pain—controlled by opioids and corticosteroids

Pain Assessment

A comprehensive pain assessment in palliative care includes a thorough history, a careful physical examination, and, in some cases, interpretation of laboratory values or imaging results (Box 1.2).[6]

While conducting a thorough history, it is useful to consider those patients at risk for inadequate assessment and management of pain (Box 1.3, Table 1.1).

Nonopioids

Acetaminophen (also called paracetamol) is analgesic and antipyretic and is found in a variety of combination prescription and over-the-counter compounds. Hepatic toxicity can result from excessive use, and a firm limit on daily consumption has not been established.[11,12] Some sources recommend no more

Box 1.1 Selected Cancer Pain Syndromes

Tumor-Related Pain Syndromes
- Bone metastases
- Hepatic capsule distention due to metastases
- Plexus involvement by tumor

Treatment-Related Pain Syndromes

Surgical-Related Pain Syndromes
- Post-amputation phantom pain
- Post-thoracotomy pain
- Post-mastectomy pain

Radiation-Related Pain Syndromes
- Chest pain/tightness
- Cystitis
- Enteritis
- Fistula formation
- Myelopathy
- Osteoporosis
- Osteoradionecrosis
- Pelvic fractures
- Peripheral nerve entrapment
- Plexopathies
- Proctitis
- Secondary malignancies

Chemotherapy-Related Pain Syndromes
- Chemotherapy-induced peripheral neuropathy
- Osteonecrosis from corticosteroids

Stem Cell Transplant–Mediated Chronic Graft versus Host Disease
- Scleroderma-like skin changes
- Eye pain and dryness
- Oral pain and reduced jaw motion
- Dysuria
- Dyspareunia, vaginal pain
- Paresthesias
- Arthralgias, myalgias

Hormonal Therapy–Related Pain Syndromes
- Osteoporotic compression fractures
- Arthralgias

Pain Unrelated to Tumor or Treatment
- Comorbid conditions, such as diabetic neuropathy, arthritis

From references 1–4.

than 2,000 mg per day, while others suggest up to 3,000 mg per day may be safe. This needs to be tailored to the patient. Altered hepatic function, excessive alcohol intake, and other comorbid factors may place some patients at elevated risk, and these individuals should be advised to avoid acetaminophen. Renal toxicity is another potential adverse effect of this agent. Acetaminophen is available in oral formulations, including liquids and suppositories, and, more recently, an injectable formulation has been used to treat pain and fever.[13]

Opioids

A wide array of opioids is available, allowing rotation when one opioid is ineffective or when it produces uncontrolled adverse effects (Box 1.5). Immediate-release agents provide faster onset for rescue when breakthrough

Box 1.2 Template for Comprehensive Pain History Documentation

Chief Report

Pain History

   Location(s), referral, radiating pattern

   Duration

   Intensity (within the last 24 hours, at rest, with movement)

   Quality

   Timing

   Aggravating/alleviating factors

   Other symptoms associated with pain

   Functional changes/interference with daily activities

Current therapies

   • Medications—duration, response

   • Radiation therapy

   • Other—nerve blocks, vertebroplasty, PT/OT, acupuncture, etc.

Prior treatment, response, adverse effects, reason for discontinuing

   • Medications—dose, duration, adverse effects

   • Radiation therapy (sites)

   • Other—nerve blocks, vertebroplasty, PT/OT, acupuncture, etc.

Past Medical History (PMH)

   The PMH includes *relevant* serious illness, chronic diseases, surgical procedures, and injuries the patient has experienced.

Social History

Substance Use History

   Smoking

   Alcohol (ETOH)

   Recreational drug use

   Family history of addictive disease

   Physical or sexual abuse, especially as preteen or teenager

Medication History

   Current medications, including prescription and nonprescription medications, name and dosage for each.

Review of Systems (ROS)

   Perform a Review of Symptoms that may occur along with pain. May use Edmonton Symptom Assessment System (ESAS) or other symptom assessment tool in place of ROS.

   GENERAL: endorses fatigue, sleep

   HEENT: xerostomia, denies dysphagia

   CV: denies chest pain

   RESP: denies SOB, cough

(continued)

Box 1.2 Continued

GI: last BM x days ago, consistency x, appetite (poor/good), nausea and vomiting

GU: denies urgency, frequency, incontinence, or dysuria

MS: denies tripping or falls

NEURO: denies neuropathy

SKIN: denies rash or open wounds

PSYCH: endorses feeling sad/depressed, finds strength through (name the focus, strategy, or intervention)

Performance Status

May use Palliative Performance Score (PPS), Eastern Cooperative Onoclogy Group (ECOG) Score, Karnofsky Score, or other tools. This helps determine function and prognosis and track change over time.

Physical Exam

List the physical assessment findings that are "remarkable" or contribute to understanding the pain experience and/or etiology.

Patient Goals

What the patient hopes to achieve if pain is relieved (e.g., return to work, play with grandchildren, go to church).

Impression/Problem List

Recommendations/Plan

pain occurs, and controlled-release products allow more constant control of pain. Various routes of administration allow personalized care when oral delivery is not feasible.

There are significant differences between opioids. Codeine is a prodrug and must be metabolized to morphine by the action of the CYP2D6 enzyme.[14,15]

Box 1.3 Groups at Risk for Inadequate Assessment and Undertreatment of Pain

- Infants and children
- Elderly
- Cognitively impaired
- Nonverbal individuals
- People with mental health disorders
- Minorities
- Non–English-speaking individuals
- Long-term survivors
- Socioeconomically disadvantaged
- Uninsured
- Those with current or past substance use disorders

From references 2, 7, 8.

Table 1.1 Assessment Tools for Special Adult Populations

Tool	Intended Population
Assessment of Discomfort in Dementia (ADD)	Dementia
Behavioral Pain Scale (BPS)	Intensive care, unresponsive adults
Checklist of Nonverbal Pain Indicators (CNPI)	Dementia
Critical Care Pain Observation Tool (CPOT)	Intensive care, unresponsive adults
Doloplus 2	Dementia, palliative care
Nursing Assistant-Administered Instrument to Assess Pain in Demented Individuals (NOPPAIN)	Dementia
Pain Assessment Scale for Seniors with Limited Ability to Communicate (PACSLAC)	Dementia
Pain Assessment in Advanced Dementia (PAINAD)	Dementia

From references 9 and 10.

Inadequate analgesia can result in patients who are poor metabolizers, whereas increased toxicity and overdose have been reported in individuals (or a breastfeeding baby) who are ultra-rapid metabolizers of this enzyme.[16,17]

Tramadol is a weak opioid agonist and a serotonin-norepinephrine reuptake inhibitor. Due to this dual action, it has a ceiling of 300 mg per day, and naloxone will not completely reverse overdose.[18] Tramadol should be avoided in patients with seizure risk or suicidal ideation. Dizziness is the most common adverse effect. Tapentadol is also an opioid agonist and norepinephrine reuptake inhibitor with little action on serotonin reuptake. Caution is warranted when adding antidepressants to either tramadol or tapentadol, since they may cause serotonin syndrome. As with tramadol, naloxone will not completely reverse the effects of overdose with tapentadol.

Methadone can be a highly effective analgesic: it may prevent or limit hyperalgesia, it appears to be useful for neuropathic pain, and it is inexpensive. Several challenges complicate the use of methadone, and several guidelines recommend a palliative care consultation when considering its use (Box 1.4, Table 1.2).

Box 1.4 Methadone Prescribing Recommendations

- Start low:
  - 10 mg or less per day in divided doses (q 8h or q 12h)
  - Regardless of whether patient is opioid naïve or tolerant
- Provide breakthrough pain medications using short acting opioids—not methadone.
- Increase no more than 25–50% weekly, generally no more often than every 3–7 days.
- Use caution when combining with benzodiazepines or other sedating drugs, especially at night.
- Use caution in patients with sleep apnea, respiratory infection.

From references 19, 20.

Table 1.2 Selected Methadone Drug–Drug Interactions

Inducers (decrease methadone levels)	Inhibitors (increase methadone levels)
• Abacavir	• Cimetidine
• Amprenavir	• Ciprofloxacin
• Barbiturates	• Diazepam
• Carbamazepine	• Diltiazem
• Cocaine	• Disulfiram
• Dexamethasone	• Fluconazole
• Efavirenz	• Grapefruit
• Heroin	• Haloperidol
• Lopinavir + Ritonavir	• Ketoconazole
• Nelfinavir	• Macrolides (erythromycin, clarithromycin)
• Nevirapine	• Metronidazole
• Phenytoin	• Omeprazole
• Rifampin	• Sorafenib
• Spironolactone	• SSRIs (fluoxetine, paroxetine, nefazodone, sertraline)
• St. John's Wort	

From references 20, 21.

Adjuvant Analgesics

Adjuvant analgesics include agents that have other purposes but have been found to be analgesic primarily in the management of neuropathic pain (Table 1.3).

Corticosteroids are highly effective in reducing the tumor burden of lymphoma. They can open airway or gastrointestinal obstructions from this malignancy. Added benefits of corticosteroids include improved appetite for

Box 1.5 Opioid Rotation/Switching Opioids

Step 1
• Calculate the equianalgesic dose using a standard table or online calculator.
• Reduce dose by 25–50% to account for incomplete cross-tolerance between opioids.

Step 2
• Consider an additional increase or decrease of 15–30% based on medical and psychosocial characteristics.
• Consider adverse effects, risk of withdrawal.
• Frequently reassess and titrate.
• Provide an oral rescue dose of 10–20% of 24-hour dose.

From references 22, 23.

Table 1.3 Adjuvant Analgesics

Drug Class	Daily Adult Starting Dose (Range)	Routes of Administration	Adverse Effects
Antidepressants	Nortriptyline 10–25 mg q hs	PO	Anticholinergic effects
	Venlafaxine 37.5 mg bid	PO	Nausea, dizziness
	Duloxetine 30 mg qd		Nausea
Antiepilepsy drugs	Gabapentin 100 mg tid	PO	Dizziness
	Pregabalin 50 mg tid	PO	Dizziness
	Clonazepam 0.5–1 mg q hs, bid or tid	PO	Sedation
Corticosteroids	Dexamethasone 2–20 mg qd	PO/IV/SQ	Steroid psychosis
			Dyspepsia
Lidocaine	Lidocaine patch 5% q day	Topical IV/SQ	Rare skin erythema
	Lidocaine infusion		Perioral numbness, Cardiac changes
N-Methyl-D-aspartic acid (NMDA) antagonists	Ketamine (see text for dosing)	PO/IV	Hallucinations

From references 2, 12, 24–28.

approximately 2 weeks which can relieve fatigue and possibly depression.[29] However, it is important to consider side effects (Box 1.6).

Lidocaine and other local anesthetics have been limited by the lack of an oral formulation. Topical solutions and patches may relieve more superficial pain syndromes. Spinal delivery, either alone or in combination with opioids and other agents, can be useful, but administration requires specialists to insert catheters and potentially complicated and/or expensive delivery

Box 1.6 Drug–Drug Interactions Involving Dexamethasone: Potential to Decrease Chemotherapy Levels

Erlotinib
Gefitinib
Ibrutinib
Lapatinib
Pazopanib
Ruxolitinib
Sorafenib
Sunitinib
Temsirolimus

systems (e.g., catheter care, external or implanted pumps). Infusions of parenteral lidocaine, particularly with intractable neuropathic pain, may be effective (Box 1.7).

Ketamine is an *N*-methyl-D-aspartic acid (NMDA) antagonist that is thought to be useful in relieving neuropathic pain, in reducing opioid doses

---

Box 1.7 Lidocaine Infusion Guidelines: Virginia Commonwealth University

Thomas Palliative Care Guidelines
Lidocaine Infusion for Severe Pain

Purpose

Lidocaine infusion has been reported as an effective intervention in individuals having refractory pain, in which opioids are not effective.

Protocol

1. Challenge and infusion: Prior to a lidocaine infusion, a lidocaine challenge is routinely done. Lidocaine 100 mg IV over a half-hour period is used. If effective (improvement in pain score), an infusion of 0.5–2 mg/kg/hour will be initiated. This infusion may be titrated by 20%/hour, not to exceed 2 mg/kg/hour. Doses above 2 mg/hour are rarely needed. Lidocaine 2,000 mg in 500 mL/D5W can be ordered to have available if the test dose is successful.

2. Monitoring: During infusion, observe and document vital signs and pain intensity every 15 minutes.

3. Goals of therapy
   a. Pain relief
   b. Decrease opioids rapidly and to the lowest dose possible; safe administration with minimal side effects

4. Side effects are rare when given in low doses. The most serious side effect is an allergic reaction.
   a. An allergic reaction may include difficulty breathing and irregular heartbeat or other signs of anaphylaxis.
   b. The common side effects are numbness around the mouth, dryness, or a sense of being intoxicated.
   c. Other potential side effects may include hives, hallucination, muscle twitches, and, in rare cases, seizures.

5. Long-term therapy may be initiated with lidocaine or mexiletine.

6. **Contraindication**: Hypersensitivity to lidocaine or other amide anesthetics (mepivacaine, prilocaine, dibucaine, and procainamide). Add precautions: bradycardia, congestive heart failure, heart block, hypovolemia, liver disease, renal impairment, shock, Wolff-Parkinson-White syndrome.

Original 2008; Reviewed April 2010, October 2012, September 2013.

Source: Ferrini R, Paice, J. How to initiate and monitor infusional lidocaine for severe and/or neuropathic pain. *J Support Oncol.* 2004; 2(1), 90–4. Available at http://www.oncologypractice.com/jso/journal/articles/0201090.pdf.

when high doses appear ineffective, or in the management of opioid-induced hyperalgesia.[30–32] Although often used in intraoperative and postoperative settings, ketamine's use in palliative care has been hampered by the lack of a commercially available preparation (Box 1.8).

Box 1.8 Ketamine Protocol for Oral or Parenteral Administration in Palliative Care

Purpose

This is an adjunct medication often considered for pain refractory to opioids or intractable side effects from opioids, particularly if the pain is neuropathic in nature or if a high degree of morphine tolerance is suspected.

Definition

Ketamine is an N-methyl-D-aspartate receptor (NMDA) agent that may be opioid-sparing.

Protocol

Oral Dosing

- The typical starting dose is 10–15 mg po q6h. Reversal of morphine tolerance may occur at low doses, whereas management of neuropathic pain is likely to require higher doses.
- There is no commercially available oral product. The injectable product may be diluted from its standard concentration of 50 mg/mL or 100 mg/mL with cherry syrup or cola to mask the bitter taste when given orally.
- Consider decreasing long-acting opioid by 25–50%.
- Dosing may be increased *daily* by 10 mg q 6h until pain is relieved or side effects occur. Do not increase doses more frequently than every 24 hours.
- Major side effects include dizziness, a dreamlike feeling, and auditory or visual hallucinations. If intolerable side effects occur, ketamine should be decreased to the previous dose or discontinued. Resolution may not occur for 24 hours.
- Oral doses as high as 1,000 mg per day have been reported in the neuropathic pain literature, with average oral doses of 200 mg per day in divided doses required for pain relief.

IV Dosing

- Ketamine may be given intravenously or subcutaneously, if the oral route is not available.
- Some facilities allow a ketamine challenge. A trial of 10 mg IV can be considered, which may be repeated in 15–30 minutes.
- The starting infusion dose of 0.2 mg/kg/hr can be increased by 0.1 mg/kg/hr q 6h, with upward titrations to 0.5 mg/kg/hr or 800 mg in 24 hrs.
- Consider decreasing long-acting opioid dose by 25–50%.
- The injectable solution is irritating, and the subcutaneous needle may need to be changed daily.
- For side effects of hallucinations or a dreamlike state, benzodiazepines can be given prophylactically or haloperidol can be given when the effects occur.

Table 1.4 Biopsychosocial Model: Nonpharmacologic Interventions

Biological	Psychological/Social/Spiritual
Disease-modifying therapies • Chemotherapy • Radiation therapy	Cognitive-behavioral therapies
Kyphoplasty/vertebroplasty	Mindfulness/Meditation
Nerve blocks	Guided imagery
Ablative procedures	Hypnosis
Physical/occupational and other rehabilitation therapies • Bracing/orthotics	Biofeedback
Exercise	Prayer
Heat/cold	Music
Massage	Art therapy
Acupuncture and other integrative procedures	Support groups
From references 33, 34–41, 42.	

Nonpharmacologic Interventions for Pain

See Table 1.4.

Safe Practices, Safe Storage, and Safe Disposal

Medications should be kept locked, not stored in the medicine cabinet or on the kitchen counter. Medications should never be shared and should be used only for pain relief. Safe disposal of medications prevents access by others (e.g., children, pets, individuals with intent to use the drugs recreationally or to sell these

---

Box 1.9 Universal Precautions

Assess

• Pain
• Risk for addiction/diversion

Opioid management agreements or "contracts": Limited evidence in palliative care

Adherence monitoring

• Urine drug testing
• Pill counts
• Prescription monitoring programs

From reference 44.

> **Box 1.10 Differential Diagnosis of Aberrant Drug-Taking Behavior**
>
> **Addiction**
> **Pseudo-addiction (inadequate analgesia)**
> - Amount of drug prescribed too low—low dose, inadequate number of tablets
> - Partial fill provided by pharmacy
> - Insurance limits, prior authorization
>
> **Other psychiatric disorders**
> - Chemical coping
> - Mood disorders (anxiety, depression)
> - Encephalopathy
> - Borderline personality disorder
>
> **Inability to follow a treatment plan**
> - Low literacy
> - Use of pain medication to treat other symptoms (sleep, anxiety, depression)
> - Misunderstanding regarding "prn" or as needed doses
> - Fear of pain returning
>
> **Criminal intent**
>
> From references 45–47.

agents) and limits impact on the environment.[43] The Environmental Protection Agency (EPA) advises against flushing medications into water systems (http://water.epa.gov/scitech/swguidance/ppcp/upload/ppcpflyer.pdf).

Safe Prescribing

Because there is no absolute predictor for who might misuse medications, chronic pain management experts recommend the use of "universal precautions" (Box 1.9). The palliative APRN should have an understanding of the elements of aberrant behavior (Box 1.10).

Conclusion

Effective pain management in palliative care requires knowledge of common pain etiologies, as well as skill in conducting a thorough assessment.

References

1. Glare PA, Davies PS, Finlay E, et al. Pain in cancer survivors. *J Clin Oncol.* 2014; 32(16): 1739–47.
2. Paice JA, Ferrell B. The management of cancer pain. *CA Cancer J Clin.* 2011; 61(3): 157–82.

3. Paice JA. Chronic treatment-related pain in cancer survivors. *Pain*. 2011; 152: S84–9.

4. Bennett MI, Rayment C, Hjermstad M, Aass N, Caraceni A, Kaasa S. Prevalence and aetiology of neuropathic pain in cancer patients: a systematic review. *Pain*. 2012; 153(2): 359–65.

5. Rayment C, Hjermstad MJ, Aass N, et al. Neuropathic cancer pain: prevalence, severity, analgesics and impact from the European Palliative Care Research Collaborative-Computerised Symptom Assessment study. *Palliat Med*. 2013; 27(8): 714–21.

6. Hui D, Bruera E. A personalized approach to assessing and managing pain in patients with cancer. *J Clin Oncol*. 2014; 32(16): 1640–6.

7. Fisch MJ, Lee JW, Weiss M, et al. Prospective, observational study of pain and analgesic prescribing in medical oncology outpatients with breast, colorectal, lung, or prostate cancer. *J Clin Oncol*. 2012; 30(16): 1980–8.

8. Kwon JH. Overcoming barriers in cancer pain management. *J Clin Oncol*. 2014; 32(16): 1727–33.

9. Bjoro K, Herr K. Assessment of pain in the nonverbal or cognitively impaired older adult. *Clin Geriatr Med*. 2008; 24(2): 237–62.

10. Herr K, Bjoro K, Decker S. Tools for assessment of pain in nonverbal older adults with dementia: a state-of-the-science review. *J Pain Symptom Manage*. 2006; 31(2): 170–92.

11. Chun LJ, Tong MJ, Busuttil RW, Hiatt JR. Acetaminophen hepatotoxicity and acute liver failure. *J Clin Gastroenterol*. 2009; 43(4): 342–9.

12. Vardy J, Agar M. Nonopioid drugs in the treatment of cancer pain. *J Clin Oncol*. 2014; 32(16): 1677–90.

13. Yeh YC, Reddy P. Clinical and economic evidence for intravenous acetaminophen. *Pharmacotherapy*. 2012; 32(6): 559–79.

14. Prommer E. Role of codeine in palliative care. *J Opioid Manag*. 2011; 7(5): 401–6.

15. Racoosin JA, Roberson DW, Pacanowski MA, Nielsen DR. New evidence about an old drug—risk with codeine after adenotonsillectomy. *N Engl J Med*. 2013; 368(23): 2155–7.

16. Bateman DN, Eddleston M, Sandilands E. Codeine and breastfeeding. *Lancet*. 2008; 372(9639): 625.

17. Madadi P, Koren G, Cairns J, et al. Safety of codeine during breastfeeding: fatal morphine poisoning in the breastfed neonate of a mother prescribed codeine. *Can Fam Physician*. 2007; 53(1): 33–5.

18. Tassinari D, Drudi F, Rosati M, Tombesi P, Sartori S, Maltoni M. The second step of the analgesic ladder and oral tramadol in the treatment of mild to moderate cancer pain: a systematic review. *Palliat Med*. 2011; 25(5): 410–23.

19. Parsons HA, de la Cruz M, El Osta B, et al. Methadone initiation and rotation in the outpatient setting for patients with cancer pain. *Cancer*. 2010; 116(2): 520–8.

20. Chou R, Cruciani RA, Fiellin DA, et al. Methadone safety: a clinical practice guideline from the American Pain Society and College on Problems of Drug Dependence, in collaboration with the Heart Rhythm Society. *J Pain*. 2014; 15(4): 321–37.

21. Kapur BM, Hutson JR, Chibber T, Luk A, Selby P. Methadone: a review of drug–drug and pathophysiological interactions. *Crit Rev Clin Lab Sci*. 2011; 48(4): 171–95.

22. Mercadante S, Caraceni A. Conversion ratios for opioid switching in the treatment of cancer pain: a systematic review. *Palliat Med.* 2011; 25(5): 504–15.

23. Swarm RA, Abernethy AP, Anghelescu DL, et al. Adult cancer pain. *J Natl Compr Canc Netw.* 2013; 11(8): 992–1022.

24. Mishra S, Bhatnagar S, Goyal GN, Rana SP, Upadhya SP. A comparative efficacy of amitriptyline, gabapentin, and pregabalin in neuropathic cancer pain: a prospective randomized double-blind placebo-controlled study. *Am J Hosp Palliat Care.* 2012; 29(3): 177–82.

25. Baron R, Brunnmuller U, Brasser M, May M, Binder A. Efficacy and safety of pregabalin in patients with diabetic peripheral neuropathy or postherpetic neuralgia: open-label, non-comparative, flexible-dose study. *Eur J Pain.* 2008; 12(7): 850–8.

26. Smith EM, Pang H, Cirrincione C, et al. Effect of duloxetine on pain, function, and quality of life among patients with chemotherapy-induced painful peripheral neuropathy: a randomized clinical trial. *JAMA.* 2013; 309(13): 1359–67.

27. Paulsen O, Aass N, Kaasa S, Dale O. Do corticosteroids provide analgesic effects in cancer patients? A systematic literature review. *J Pain Symptom Manage.* 2013; 46(1): 96–105.

28. Saarto T, Wiffen PJ. Antidepressants for neuropathic pain: a Cochrane review. *J Neurol Neurosurg Psychiatry.* 2010; 81(12): 1372–3.

29. Yennurajalingam S, Frisbee-Hume S, Palmer JL, et al. Reduction of cancer-related fatigue with dexamethasone: a double-blind, randomized, placebo-controlled trial in patients with advanced cancer. *J Clin Oncol.* 2013; 31(25): 3076–82.

30. Okamoto Y, Tsuneto S, Tanimukai H, et al. Can gradual dose titration of ketamine for management of neuropathic pain prevent psychotomimetic effects in patients with advanced cancer? *Am J Hosp Palliat Care.* 2013; 30(5): 450–4.

31. Bell RF, Eccleston C, Kalso EA. Ketamine as an adjuvant to opioids for cancer pain. *Cochrane Database Syst Rev.* 2012; 11: CD003351.

32. Bredlau AL, Thakur R, Korones DN, Dworkin RH. Ketamine for pain in adults and children with cancer: a systematic review and synthesis of the literature. *Pain Med.* 2013; 14(10): 1505–17.

33. Thomas ML, Elliott JE, Rao SM, Fahey KF, Paul SM, Miaskowski C. A randomized, clinical trial of education or motivational-interviewing-based coaching compared to usual care to improve cancer pain management. *Oncol Nurs Forum.* 2012; 39(1): 39–49.

34. Kwekkeboom KL, Cherwin CH, Lee JW, Wanta B. Mind-body treatments for the pain-fatigue-sleep disturbance symptom cluster in persons with cancer. *J Pain Symptom Manage.* 2010; 39(1): 126–38.

35. Collinge W, MacDonald G, Walton T. Massage in supportive cancer care. *Semin Oncol Nurs.* 2012; 28(1): 45–54.

36. Toth M, Marcantonio ER, Davis RB, Walton T, Kahn JR, Phillips RS. Massage therapy for patients with metastatic cancer: a pilot randomized controlled trial. *J Altern Complement Med.* 2013; 19(7): 650–6.

37. Greer JA, Traeger L, Bemis H, et al. A pilot randomized controlled trial of brief cognitive-behavioral therapy for anxiety in patients with terminal cancer. *Oncologist.* 2012; 17(10): 1337–45.

38. Balboni MJ, Babar A, Dillinger J, et al. "It depends": viewpoints of patients, physicians, and nurses on patient-practitioner prayer in the setting of advanced cancer. *J Pain Symptom Manage.* 2011; 41(5): 836–47.

39. Sharp DM, Walker MB, Chaturvedi A, et al. A randomised, controlled trial of the psychological effects of reflexology in early breast cancer. *Eur J Cancer*. 2010; 46(2): 312–22.

40. Cheville AL, Basford JR. Role of rehabilitation medicine and physical agents in the treatment of cancer-associated pain. *J Clin Oncol*. 2014; 32(16): 1691–702.

41. Alemann G, Kastler A, Barbe DA, Aubry S, Kastler B. Treatment of painful extraspinal bone metastases with percutaneous bipolar radiofrequency under local anesthesia: feasibility and efficacy in twenty-eight cases. *J Palliat Med*. 2014; 17(8): 947–52.

42. Syrjala KL, Jensen MP, Mendoza ME, Yi JC, Fisher HM, Keefe FJ. Psychological and behavioral approaches to cancer pain management. *J Clin Oncol*. 2014; 32(16): 1703–11.

43. Okie S. A flood of opioids, a rising tide of deaths. *N Engl J Med*. 2010; 363(21): 1981–5.

44. Starrels JL, Becker WC, Alford DP, Kapoor A, Williams AR, Turner BJ. Systematic review: treatment agreements and urine drug testing to reduce opioid misuse in patients with chronic pain. *Ann Intern Med*. 2010; 152(11): 712–20.

45. Chou R, Fanciullo GJ, Fine PG, et al. Clinical guidelines for the use of chronic opioid therapy in chronic noncancer pain. *J Pain*. 2009; 10(2): 113–30.

46. Kircher S, Zacny J, Apfelbaum SM, et al. Understanding and treating opioid addiction in a patient with cancer pain. *J Pain*. 2011; 12(10): 1025–31.

47. Cheatle MD, O'Brien CP, Mathai K, Hansen M, Grasso M, Yi P. Aberrant behaviors in a primary care-based cohort of patients with chronic pain identified as misusing prescription opioids. *J Opioid Manag*. 2013; 9(5): 315–24.

Chapter 2

Dyspnea

Kathleen Broglio

Key Points

- Dyspnea is a prevalent sensory/affective symptom that affects individuals with advanced disease(s) and often worsens toward the end of life.
- A dyspnea assessment using a biopsychosocial approach, with the understanding that dyspnea affects the entire person, should be completed.
- A multimodal (pharmacologic, nonpharmacologic, and psychoeducational) approach to dyspnea management should be implemented.

Definition

Descriptive qualities of dyspnea have been separated into three categories (air hunger, work, and tightness).[1] Descriptions of dyspnea in those with chronic obstructive pulmonary disease (COPD) and heart disease have been clustered into categories describing the rate and depth of breathing, obstructive or restrictive qualities, effort or work of breathing, or feelings of distress.[2,3] Descriptors include "frightening," "worried," "depressed," and "awful"; "air hunger," "breathlessness," "gasping," "exhaustion,"[4] "not enough air," "short of breath," "suffocation," "choking," and "drowning."[5] There are many causes of dyspnea in advanced illness (Table 2.1).

Pathophysiology and Mechanisms of Dyspnea

It is generally accepted that dyspnea emanates from changes in activity in central chemoreceptors.[6] Both hypercapnia and hypoxia can induce a sense of "air hunger" independent of changes in respiratory activity.[7] Changes in mechanoreceptor activity in the lung, chest wall, upper airway, and facial receptors can also contribute to dyspnea.[6] It has been hypothesized that changes within the airway itself and the associated activity of pulmonary receptors generate a sense of tightness and constant respiratory discomfort.[8] Dyspnea can arise from an increased sense of the work of breathing in those with fatigue, weakened respiratory muscles, or obstructive diseases.[6,9] Neuromechanical dissociation, a mismatch between incoming information

Table 2.1 Potential Causes of Dyspnea in Advanced Disease[a]

Pulmonary	Cardiac	Systemic	Treatment-related	Psychological
Airway obstructions	Congestive heart failure (CHF)	Cachexia	Surgical	Anxiety
Carcinomatosis	Ischemia	Steroid myopathy	• Lobectomy	Panic
Chest wall infiltrations	Pericardial effusion	Hepatomegaly	• Pneumonectomy	
Chronic obstructive pulmonary disease (COPD)	Pulmonary hypertension	Ascites	Chemotherapy	
Interstitial lung disease		Anemia	• Pulmonary or cardiac toxicity	
		Metabolic abnormalities	Radiation side effects	
Effusions		Obesity	• Pneumonitis	
Embolism		Hyperventilation	• Fibrosis	
Pneumonia		Neuromuscular abnormalities	• Pericarditis	
Pneumothorax				
Superior vena cava obstruction				
Tumor				

[a]Only partial list of more common causes. Adapted from Chan et al., 2010. Ref 10.

> **Box 2.1 Potential Mechanisms for Dyspnea**
>
> **Central Chemoreceptor Changes**
> - Hypoxia
> - Hypercapnia
>
> **Mechanoreceptor Stimulation**
> - Lung, chest wall, upper airway, facial area
>
> **Respiratory Muscle Effort**
> - Increased sense of breathing due to fatigue/obstructive processes
>
> **Neuromechanical Disassociation**
> - Mismatch between respiratory and brain command center

from the respiratory system and outgoing commands from the brain center, can also cause dyspnea[6, 9] (Box 2.1).

Clinical Assessment

A biopsychosocial assessment is imperative because the individual's experience and interpretation of dyspnea and preferences for treatment may vary and change with disease progression.[10]

Further diagnostic testing should be guided by the goals of care and the added value of information gleaned from diagnostic outcomes on treatment or change in outcome (see Box 2.2).

Management

Although there has been progress made in understanding the mechanisms of dyspnea, the treatment of dyspnea has not progressed significantly[11] (Table 2.2).

Pharmacologic Management

First-Line Therapy: Opioids

Dyspnea has been compared to pain in terms of the need to address it as a basic human right for treatment—the evidence is there for opioid therapy, and to deny it is to deny a human right.[12] Opioids are the first-line treatment for dyspnea.[11,13] Opioids may reduce dyspnea by decreasing the respiratory drive, by altering responses to hypoxia and hypercapnia, and through changes in bronchoconstriction.[14] Morphine, the most widely studied opioid, has been shown to be effective for dyspnea.[15–17]

Box 2.2 Assessment of Dyspnea

Clinical Interview

- PQRST (**P**rovoking/palliating factors, **Q**uality/characteristic, **R**elation to other symptoms such as anxiety, fatigue and pain, **S**everity, **T**iming)
- Use of disease-modifying therapies that affect respiratory system when indicated
- Lifestyle factors—smoke exposure

Selected Assessment Tools[a]

Unidimensional tools—measure severity
- Modified BORG dyspnea rating scale
- Visual analogue scale (VAS)
- Numeric rating

Patient self-assessment tools in advanced disease—measure severity of multiple symptoms
- Memorial Symptom Assessment Scale (MSAS)
- Edmonton Symptom Assessment System (ESAS)

Disease-specific tools—address physical/affective components
- Dyspneoea-12 (COPD, heart failure, interstitial lung disease)
- Cancer Dyspnea Scale (CDS)

Observation scale—for patients unable to report
- Respiratory Distress Observation Scale (RDOS)

Physical Examination

- General—pallor, cachexia, ascites, edema
- Respiratory—respiratory rate, oxygen saturation, breathing pattern, breath sounds
- Cardiac—pulse rate, heart sounds, jugular venous pressure

Laboratory—Diagnostic Testing[b]

- Hemoglobin, oxygen saturation, pCO_2, basic metabolic panel
- Chest x-ray
- CT or perfusion scans, echocardiograms

[a]There are many more tools than are listed; no specific one is endorsed for use by the American Thoracic Society or the American College of Chest Physicians.

[b]Depends on goals of care.

Opioids are still underused due to fears about respiratory depression.[11,13] Results from studies of patients with COPD,[16,18] cancer,[16,19] or heart failure[20] evaluating the use of opioids for dyspnea failed to demonstrate a relationship between opioids and respiratory compromise. The proposed doses of morphine for opioid-naïve adult patients with dyspnea range from 0.5 to 1 mg orally q 4h[21] to 5 to 10 mg orally q 3–4h[22] to 10 mg of extended-release oral morphine

Table 2.2 Selected Treatment Options for Dyspnea in Advanced Disease

Intervention	Comment
Pharmacologic Opioids (IV, SC, PO)	First-line treatment for dyspnea related to cancer, COPD; efficacy in CHF not determined.
	Optimal dosing has not been determined. Starting morphine doses range from 0.5 to 10 mg orally q 4h; other opioids may also be effective if morphine is contraindicated.
Benzodiazepines	Not first-line recommendation, but potentially useful for dyspnea refractory to other measures or in dyspnea-associated anxiety
Furosemide	Oral and intravenous furosemide may be helpful in CHF. Nebulized furosemide may be useful in COPD.
Oxygen	Beneficial for hypoxemia; may be beneficial for those not hypoxemic; trial is warranted.
Noninvasive ventilation	May be useful for exacerbations of COPD and in those with hypercapnia
Interventional Pleurodesis	May decrease dyspnea due to pleural effusions
Tunneled catheter	May decrease dyspnea due to pleural effusions
Bronchial stenting	May decrease dyspnea secondary to obstructions
Nonpharmacologic Rehabilitation	Breathing training—COPD
	Pulmonary rehabilitation—efficacy in COPD, some evidence in cancer
Psychoeducational	Counseling, education, relaxation, Internet-based self-management—may increase self-efficacy
Fans	Low-risk treatment, may be beneficial
Acupuncture	Equivocal evidence

daily with titration to 30 mg/day for chronic dyspnea.[16] A similar approach to that of pain management should be employed: "start low and go slow." There is an exception, however, when managing dyspnea toward the end of life. In an acute care setting, opioids may be given intravenously and the dose titrated up rapidly. The dose should be adjusted for those who are older and frail with multiple comorbidities.

Nebulized opioids may be attractive to individuals who may not want to take oral medications.[23] Results from studies of nebulized morphine were equivocal, whereas those from studies of hydromorphone and fentanyl showed possible benefit in those with cancer.[24]

Second-Line Therapy: Benzodiazepines

Benzodiazepines have been used for dyspnea and may treat the affective response to dyspnea. However, in a systematic review of benzodiazepines for dyspnea, the analysis from seven studies in advanced cancer and COPD did not show a significant benefit regardless of type, dose, or route.[25] Anxiolytics (including benzodiazepines) have not been recommended by the American and Canadian thoracic societies for dyspnea in patients with COPD.[11,26]

However, benzodiazepines have been shown to be effective in some recent small studies.[5,27,28]

Benzodiazepines may be used for dyspnea refractory to opioids or other nonpharmacologic measures, although quality studies are needed to further evaluate their potential efficacy.[25] Lorazepam is recommended due to its relatively short half-life and availability in liquid form.[28] Dosing can start as low as 0.25 mg orally or sublingually q 4h. Individuals with significant anxiety who may not be approaching the end of life may benefit from treatment of anxiety with agents such as selective serotonin reuptake inhibitors.

Oxygen Therapy

Oxygen is generally the first treatment clinicians consider when someone is dyspneic. The use of oxygen is warranted if dyspnea is related to a physiologic event limiting the delivery of necessary oxygen to the body, such as for those with COPD. However, in advanced disease, the oxygen saturation and carbon dioxide status may not correlate with the perception of dyspnea. For studies on the pros and cons of oxygen therapy, see the companion volume to this book, *Advanced Practice Palliative Nursing* (2016), Chapter 24: Dyspnea. A time-limited trial of oxygen therapy to evaluate the response in dyspneic individuals with advanced disease who are not hypoxemic or only mildly hypoxemic may be an appropriate response.

Noninvasive ventilation has been studied in those with acute exacerbations of COPD. Noninvasive ventilation may provide benefit for those with advanced disease and dyspnea, but further research is needed to evaluate its efficacy in different disease states.[30] The treatment of dyspnea related to motor neuron diseases poses additional challenges because individuals must make decisions related to the use of both noninvasive and invasive ventilation not only to manage dyspnea, but also to prolong life.

Interventional Therapy

Referrals for interventional therapies to reduce dyspnea, if consistent with goals of care, may be appropriate. Mechanical or chemical pleurodesis may reduce dyspnea secondary to pleural effusions. For those with more advanced disease, the placement of a tunneled catheter for management of pleural effusions may be the most effective option.[31,32] Disease-modifying therapies, such as chemotherapy and radiation therapy, should be explored as first-line treatments for obstructions secondary to tumor burden.[33] Those with malignant airway obstructions may benefit from interventional bronchoscopy and/ or stenting.[34] However, the increased risk of infection secondary to stenting should be balanced against the possible benefit.

Nonpharmacologic Management

Treatment for dyspnea is best managed using a multimodal approach. When considering the inclusion of nonpharmacologic treatment, it is important to consider individual beliefs, the perceived relevance, insurance coverage, short-term benefits, convenience in administration, and caregiver involvement.[35]

Additional Therapies

Breathing training techniques,[26,36] the use of mobility aids,[26] and the use of neuromuscular electrical muscle stimulation[26,36] have been beneficial for dyspnea in those with COPD, but access may be limited by insurance issues. Pulmonary rehabilitation should be considered with patients with COPD and cancer.[37]

Psychoeducational Interventions

Counseling, education, and relaxation techniques to manage breathlessness have been beneficial in individuals with lung cancer.[38]

Fans

The use of portable and handheld fans has been advocated for the relief of dyspnea. It has been hypothesized that cool air on the nasoreceptors decreases the subjective feeling of dyspnea. Due to its low risk and cost, a trial of a fan is warranted except for those with facial pain secondary to trigeminal neuralgia or a neuropathic process that may be aggravated by the air movement on the face.

Dyspnea Management at the End of Life

Dyspnea may worsen in both pulmonary and nonpulmonary disease states toward the end of life. In the acute care setting, the use of an opioid infusion may treat both dyspnea and pain and may be rapidly titrated. Benzodiazepines in combination with opioids may improve moderate to severe dyspnea.[19,28] In home care settings, use of sublingual or rectal routes for opioids and benzodiazepines may alleviate dyspnea at the end of life. For a select few who experience intractable dyspnea, the use of palliative sedation may be a consideration if dyspnea cannot be controlled with opioids and benzodiazepines. See the companion volume to this book, *Advanced Practice Palliative Nursing* (2016), Chapter 51: Palliative Sedation.

Conclusion

The effective treatment of dyspnea combines the optimal treatment of the underlying pathology (when appropriate) and the associated distress. Pharmacologic and nonpharmacologic approaches can decrease dyspnea and its associated distress. Further research is necessary to optimize understanding and treatment of dyspnea. Palliative APRNs play key roles in contributing to the further development of this evidence base.

References

1. Lansing RW, Gracely RH, Banzett RB. The multiple dimensions of dyspnea: review and hypotheses. *Respir Physiol Neurobiol.* 2009; 167(1): 53–60. doi: 10.1016/j.resp.2008.07.012

2. Caroci, AS, Lareau SC. Descriptors of dyspnea by patients with chronic obstructive pulmonary disease versus congestive heart failure. *Heart Lung*. 2004; 33(2): 102–10.

3. von Leupoldt A, Balewski S, Petersen S, et al. Verbal descriptors of dyspnea in patients with COPD at different intensity levels of dyspnea. *Chest*. 2007; 132(1): 141–7.

4. Williams M, Cafarella P, Olds T, Petkov J, Frith P. The language of breathlessness differentiates between patients with COPD and age-matched adults. *Chest*. 2008; 134(3): 489–96. doi: 10.1378/chest.07-2916

5. Navigante AH, Castro MA, Cerchietti LC. Morphine versus midazolam as upfront therapy to control dyspnea perception in cancer patients while its underlying cause is sought or treated. *J Pain Symptom Manage*. 2010; 39: 820–30.

6. Chan K, Tse DMW, Sham MMK, Thorsen AB. Palliative medicine in malignant respiratory diseases. In: Hanks G, Fallon M, Cherny NI, Christakis NA, Portenoy RK, Kaasa S, eds. *Oxford Textbook of Palliative Medicine*. 4th ed. New York: Oxford University Press; 2010.

7. Moosavi SH, Golestanian E, Binks AP, Lansing RW, Brown R, Banzett RB. Hypoxic and hypercapnic drives to breathe generate equivalent levels of air hunger in humans. *J Appl Physiol*. 2003; 94(1): 141–54.

8. Binks AP, Moosavi SH, Banzett RB, Schwartzstein RM. "Tightness" sensation of asthma does not arise from the work of breathing. *Am J Respir Crit Care Med*. 2002; 165(1): 78–82.

9. Nishino T. Dyspnoea: underlying mechanisms and treatment. *Br J Anaesth*. 2011; 106(4): 463–74. doi: 10.1093/bja/aer040

10. Gysels M, Higginson IJ. The lived experience of breathlessness and its implications for care: a qualitative comparison in cancer, COPD, heart failure and MND. *BMC Palliat Care*. 2011; 10: 15.

11. Parshall MB, Schwartzsein RM, Adams L, et al. An official American Thoracic Society statement: update on the mechanisms, assessment, and management of dyspnea. *Am J Respir Critic Care Med*. 2012; 185(4): 435–52.

12. Currow DC, Abernethy AP, Ko DN. The active identification and management of chronic refractory breathlessness is a human right. *Thorax*. 2014; 69(4): 393–4. doi: 10.1136/thoraxjnl-2013-204701

13. Mahler DA, Selecky PA, Harrod CG, et al. American College of Chest Physicians consensus statement on the management of dyspnea in patients with advanced lung or heart disease. *Chest*. 2010; 137: 674–91.

14. Horton R,G. What is the role of opioids in treatment of refractory dyspnea in advanced chronic pulmonary disease? In: Goldstein NE, Morrison RS, eds. *Evidence-Based Practice of Palliative Medicine*. Philadelphia, PA: Elsevier; 2013:111–9.

15. Ben-Aharon I, Gafter-Gvili A, Leibovici L, Stemmer SM. Interventions for alleviating cancer-related dyspnea: a systematic review and meta-analysis. *Acta Oncol*. 2012; 51(8): 996–1008. doi: 10.3109/0284186X.2012.709638

16. Currow DC, McDonald C, Oaten S. et al. Once-daily opioids for chronic dyspnea: a dose increment and pharmacolvigilance study. *J Pain Symptom Manage*. 2011; 42(3): 388–99.

17. Currow DC, Quinn S, Greene A, Bull J, Johnson MJ, Abernethy AP. The longitudinal pattern of response when morphine is used to treat chronic refractory dyspnea. *J Palliat Med*. 2013; 16(8): 881–6. doi: 10.1089/jpm.2012.0591

18. Ekström MP, Bornefalk-Hermansson A, Abernethy AP, Currow DC. Safety of benzodiazepines and opioids in very severe respiratory disease: national prospective study. *BMJ*. 2014; 348: g445. doi: 10.1136/bmj.g445

19. Clemens KE, Quednau I, Klaschik E. Is there a higher risk of respiratory depression in opioid-naïve palliative care patients during symptomatic therapy of dyspnea with strong opioids? *J Palliat Med*. 2008; 11(2): 204–16. doi: 10.1089/jpm.2007.0131

20. Oxberry SG, Torgerson DJ, Bland JM, Clark AL, Cleland JG, Johnson MJ. Short-term opioids for breathlessness in stable chronic heart failure: a randomized controlled trial. *Eur J Heart Fail*. 2011; 13(9): 1006–12. doi: 10.1093/eurjhf/hfr068

21. Rocker G, Horton R, Currow D, Goodridge D, Young J, Booth S. Palliation of dyspnoea in advanced COPD: revisiting a role for opioids. *Thorax*. 2009; 64(10): 910–5. doi: 10.1136/thx.2009.116699.

22. Lanken PN, Terry PB, Delisser HM, et al. An official American Thoracic Society clinical policy statement: palliative care for patients with respiratory diseases and critical illnesses. *Am J Respir Crit Care Med*. 2008; 177(8): 912–27. doi: 10.1164/rccm.200605-587ST

23. Bausewein C, Simon S. Inhaled nebulized and intranasal opioids for the relief of breathlessness. *Curr Opin Support Palliat Care*. 2014; 8(3): 208–12. doi: 10.1097/SPC.0000000000000071

24. Boyden JY, Connor SR, Otolorin L, Nathan SD, Fine PG, Davis MS, Muir JC. Nebulized medications for the treatment of dyspnea: a literature review. *J Aerosol Med Pulm Drug Deliv*. 2014 June 10. [Epub ahead of print]

25. Simon ST, Higginson IJ, Booth S, Harding R, Bausewein C. Benzodiazepines for the relief of breathlessness in advanced malignant and non-malignant diseases in adults. *Cochrane Database Syst Rev*. 2010; (1): CD007354.

26. Marciniuk DD, Goodridge D, Hernandez P, et al. Managing dyspnea in patients with advanced chronic obstructive pulmonary disease: a Canadian Thoracic Society clinical practice guideline. *Can Respir J*. 2011; 18(2): 69–78.

27. Clemens KE, Klaschik E. Dyspnoea associated with anxiety-symptomatic therapy with opioids in combination with lorazepam and its effect on ventilation in palliative care patients. *Support Care Cancer*. 2011; 19: 2027–33. doi: 10.1007/s00520-010-1058-8

28. Gomutbutra P, O'Riordan DL, Pantilat SZ. Management of moderate-to-severe dyspnea in hospitalized patients receiving palliative care. *J Pain Symptom Manage*. 2013; 45(4): 885–91. doi: 10.1016/j.jpainsymman.2012.05.004

29. Quill TE, Bower KA, Holloway RG, et al. Dyspnea. In: *Primer of Palliative Care*. 6th ed. Chicago, IL: American Academy of Hospice and Palliative Medicine; 2014:52.

30. Gifford AH. Noninvasive ventilation as a palliative measure. *Curr Opin Support Palliat Care*. 2014; 8(3): 218–24. doi: 10.1097/SPC.0000000000000068

31. Monsky WL, Yoneda KY, MacMillan J, et al. Peritoneal and pleural ports for management of refractory ascites and pleural effusions: assessment of impact on patient quality of life and hospice/home nursing care. *J Palliat Med*. 2009; 12(9): 811–7. doi: 10.1089/jpm.2009.0061

32. Olden AM, Holloway R. Treatment of malignant pleural effusion: PleuRx catheter or talc pleurodesis? A cost-effectiveness analysis. *J Palliat Med*. 2010; 13(1): 59–65. doi: 10.1089/jpm.2009.0220

33. Grosu HB, Eapen GA, Morice RC, et al. Stents are associated with increased risk of respiratory infections in patients undergoing airway interventions

for malignant airways disease. *Chest*. 2013; 144(2): 441–9. doi: 10.1378/chest.12-1721

34. Casal RF. Update in airway stents. *Curr Opin Pulm Med*. 2010; 16(4): 321–8. doi: 10.1097/MCP.0b013e32833a260

35. Ellis J, Wagland R, Tishelman C. et al. Considerations in developing and delivering a nonpharmacological intervention for symptom management in lung cancer: the views of patients and informal caregivers. *J Pain Symptom Manage*. 2012; 44(6): 831–42. doi: 10.1016/j.jpainsymman.2011.12.274

36. Bausewein C, Booth S, Gysels M, Higginson IJ. Non-pharmacological interventions for breathlessness in advanced stages of malignant and non-malignant diseases. *Cochrane Database Syst Rev*. 2008; 2: CD005623. doi: 10.1002/14651858.CD005623.pub3

37. Lacasse Y, Martin S, Lasserson TJ, Goldstein RS. Meta-analysis of respiratory rehabilitation in chronic obstructive pulmonary disease. A Cochrane systematic review. *Eura Medicophys*. 2007; 43(4): 475–85.

38. Chan CW, Richardson A, Richardson J. Managing symptoms in patients with advanced lung cancer during radiotherapy: results of a psychoeducational randomized controlled trial. *J Pain Symptom Manage*. 2011; 41(2): 347–57. doi: 10.1016/j. jpainsymman.2010.04.024

Chapter 3

Bowel Symptoms: Constipation, Diarrhea, and Obstruction

Kimberly Chow and Lauren Koranteng

Key Points

- Constipation, diarrhea, and malignant bowel obstruction are highly prevalent and distressful symptoms in advanced illness.
- Bowel symptoms do not occur in isolation from other symptoms, and proper management requires a global understanding of the patient's experience.

Constipation

Constipation remains a largely subjective symptom that is often quantified by individuals based on what they perceive to be their normal bowel function.[1,2] Four suggested domains for diagnosis are (1) life-long history of constipation using the Rome Criteria; (2) clinical changes causing or exacerbating constipation; (3) subjective symptoms, including bloating or incomplete defecation; and (4) objective changes, such as frequency and consistency of stools.[3] Constipation is a highly distressing symptom for patients, families, and providers and can lead to a multitude of physical signs and symptoms, including anorexia, nausea, vomiting, abdominal pain, distention, and obstruction.[4–6]

The American Gastroenterology Association defines constipation as "difficult or infrequent passage of stool, at times associated with straining or a feeling of incomplete defecation."[7,8] The identification and management of constipation in palliative care have historically been complicated by the lack of a universal definition as well as by disparities between patient and provider opinions.[1–3]

Pathophysiology

Potential causes of constipation may be related to structure, disease, or personal factors and are grouped into primary or secondary causes.[9–12] Primary (e.g., idiopathic or functional) constipation occurs without an identifiable underlying cause.[7,8,11] Gastrointestinal motility is often intact, with reports of

---

Box 3.1 Secondary Causes of Constipation

- Medications (e.g., opioids, anticholinergics)
- Personal factors (e.g., time, privacy, diet, activity, fluid intake)
- Endocrine/metabolic disorders (e.g., diabetes, hypercalcemia, hypothyroidism)
- Cancer-related (e.g., tumor obstruction, spinal cord compression, electrolyte imbalances, cerebral tumors)
- Neurologic disease (e.g., cerebrovascular disease, Parkinson's disease)
- Psychological disorders (e.g., anxiety, depression, somatization)

From references 6, 7, 9, 13–15.

---

difficulty evacuating, hard stools, or dysfunction of the pelvic floor muscles or anal sphincter.[7]

Secondary causes of constipation are the result of medications, personal factors, or disorders that may be structural, metabolic, or neurologic in nature. In advanced illness, constipation is often multifactorial, caused by decreased activity, anorexia, polypharmacy, older age, side effects of disease and treatment, and psychological effects of disease (Box 3.1). Current recommendations support treating the multiple contributing factors rather than single risk factors with regard to common etiologies.[6,13]

Assessment

A subjective assessment requires a thorough history of current and past bowel patterns.[16]

The APRN may want to consider the elements of the Constipation Assessment Scale (CAS), a quick, reliable, and validated tool commonly used in palliative care. It assesses for eight symptoms that measure the severity of constipation: (1) abdominal distention or bloating, (2) change in amount of gas passed rectally, (3) less frequent bowel movements, (4) oozing liquid stool, (5) rectal fullness or pressure, (6) rectal pain with bowel movements, (7) smaller stool size, and (8) urge but inability to pass stool. [9,16–18] Medication reconciliation can help the APRN to identify common medications that may contribute to constipation (Table 3.1).

When conducting a physical exam, the APRN should always be mindful of privacy and cultural sensitivity.[14,16] Assessment includes looking for oral lesions and thrush, which can affect diet and nutrition. The abdomen should be assessed for bowel sounds, distention, tenderness, and organomegaly. Fecal masses may be palpable on rectal exam.[12] Unless the patient is immunocompromised, rectal exams help rule out fecal impaction, impaired sphincter tone, anal fissures, tumor, and/or hemorrhoids.[16]

Further workup of constipation should be dictated by life expectancy and goals of care (Box 3.2), because results may lead to unintended findings that can complicate the clinical picture and prolong the hospital stay. Table 3.2 lists laboratory studies and radiologic imaging to consider.[14,17]

Table 3.1 Drugs/Drug Classes Associated with Constipation

Drugs/Drug Class	Examples
Antacids	Calcium carbonate
Anticonvulsants	Carbamazepine, oxcarbazepine, phenobarbital
Antidepressants	Amitriptyline, doxepin
Antihistamines	Diphenhydramine
Antiparkinsonian agents	Benztropine, bromocriptine
Barium sulfate	
Calcium channel antagonists	Verapamil
Cholestyramine	
Clonidine	
Diuretics	Furosemide, hydrochlorothiazide
Nonsteroidal anti-inflammatory drugs	Ibuprofen, naproxen
Opioids	Morphine, hydromorphone
Serotonin receptor antagonists	Ondansetron, granisetron
Phenothiazines	Promethazine
Polystyrene sodium sulfonate	
Vinca alkaloids	Vincristine

From references 9, 12, 19, 20.

Management

Pharmacologic Management

Optimal pharmacologic management of constipation involves a combination of effective and appropriate prophylactic and treatment doses.[5,22] Table 3.3 offers prophylactic options to consider. The choice of agents is influenced by factors like cost, patient preference, availability, and side effects.

New studies on constipation in advanced disease have been conducted. A recent, prospective, randomized, controlled-trial demonstrated that docusate plus sennosides was no more efficacious than sennosides alone, in managing constipation in hospice patients. Tables 3.4 and 3.5 list the various classes of

Box 3.2 Differential Diagnosis of Constipation

- Psychological disorders (e.g., anxiety, depression)
- Irritable bowel syndrome
- Colonic obstruction (e.g., malignant, nonmalignant)
- Surgical adhesions
- Electrolyte imbalance
- Ileus
- Spinal cord compression

From references 12, 19.

Table 3.2 Additional Constipation Assessment Measures

Laboratory Workup	Radiologic Exam
• Complete blood count (CBC)	Abdominal radiograph (x-ray)
• Thyroid-stimulating hormone (TSH)	• Rules out obstruction
• Calcium (Ca)	• Differentiates between stool and tumor
• Serum creatinine (Cr)	• Provides very little definitive information

From references 12, 19, 21.

laxatives and bowel preparations, initial and maximum daily doses, and special considerations.

Diarrhea

Diarrhea has commonly been classified as an increase in stool frequency and liquidity; for the majority of the general population, it is self-limited and does not require medical attention.[19] The objective definition is the passage of three or more unformed stools within a 24-hour period.[32] Acute diarrhea occurs within 24–48 hours of exposure to the offending agent or event and usually subsides within 1–2 weeks.[9,19,33] Most cases have a short duration and are infectious in nature. Onset of chronic diarrhea may not occur immediately and can persist for more than 30 days.[33]

Subjectively, patients may describe any change in stool frequency, volume, or consistency as diarrhea; this should be clarified. When bowel movements are intense and variable, patients may have discomfort, anxiety, and experience social isolation. Uncontrolled, persistent diarrhea can cause increased weakness, malnutrition, dehydration, and electrolyte imbalances that may be debilitating and even life-threatening.

Table 3.3 Options for Prophylactic Management of Constipation

Start with a basic regimen based on the patient's status and preference and titrate to effect.	
Patients on opioid therapy should be on constipation prophylaxis unless contraindicated:	
Option 1	Senna 17.2 mg at bedtime or 17.2 mg oral (PO) twice daily if taking opioids.
	Consider stool softener: docusate 100 mg PO twice daily if indicated.
Option 2	Polyethylene glycol 17 g PO once daily
Option 3	Lactulose 30 mL PO once or twice daily
Option 4	Bisacodyl 1 tablet PO once daily

From references 20, 23, 24.

Table 3.4 Medications for Constipation

Generic Name (Brand Name)	Initial Dose (Init)	Comments
Bulk-Forming Agents—Absorb liquid in the GI tract and increase the bulk consistency of stool. Not recommended if unable to tolerate large volume of liquids.		
Psyllium (Metamucil)	Init: 2.5 g PO 1–3 times daily	• Drink with 8 ounces of liquid. • Separate dose by at least 2 hrs from other medications. • Onset of action: 12–72 hrs
Methylcellulose (Citrucel)	Init: 2 g 1–3 times daily as needed MDD: 6 g	• Use caution in dehydrated patients. • Onset of action: 24–48 hrs
Stimulant Laxatives—Stimulate myenteric plexus and initiate peristaltic activity and inhibit water absorption		
Senna (Senokot)	Init: 17.2 mg PO at bedtime MDD: 68.8 mg	• Previously used in combination with docusate • May cause cramping • Onset of action: 6–12 hrs
Bisacodyl (Dulcolax)	Init: 5 mg PO or 1 suppository or enema (10 mg) PR once daily MDD: 15 mg PO	• May cause cramping • Onset of action: 6–8 hrs (oral); 0.25–1 hr after rectal administration
Castor oil (Emulsoil)	Init: 15–60 mL PO once daily as needed MDD: 60 mL	• May cause cramping • Onset of action: 2–6 hrs
Surfactant/Detergent Laxatives—Lower surface tension of stool to allow mixing of aqueous and fatty substances; alter intestinal mucosal permeability		
Docusate salts (Colace)	Init: 50–300 mg PO in single or divided doses MDD: 240 mg PO for docusate calcium; 360 mg PO or docusate sodium	• Onset of action: 24–72 hrs • New study suggests no significant benefit of docusate with sennosides and to consider use on an individual basis.

(continued)

Table 3.4 Continued

Generic Name (Brand Name)	Initial Dose (Init)	Comments
Osmotic Laxatives—Cause fluid retention, distending the colon to increase peristalsis		
Lactulose (Kristalose, Chronulac, Constulose, Enulose)	Init: 15–30 mL once daily MDD: variable	• Mix with beverage to improve flavor • Costly • May cause flatulence and cramping • Onset of action: 24–48 hrs
Sorbitol	Init: 30–45 mL (27–40 g) PO once daily MDD: 45 mL PO; 120 mL PR	• Less expensive than lactulose • May cause abdominal pain, cramping, and diarrhea • Onset of action: 0.25–1 hr
Magnesium citrate (Citroma)	Init: 150–300 mL PO as a single or divided dose MDD: 300 mL PO as a laxative	• Chill to improve taste • May cause cramping • Onset of action: 3–6 hrs
Magnesium hydroxide (Milk of Magnesia)	Init: 15–60 mL PO daily, preferably at bedtime MDD: 60 mL	• May dilute with water prior to administration • Onset of action: 0.5–8 hrs
Magnesium sulfate (Epsom Salt)	Init: 10–30 g PO as single or divided doses MDD: NA	• Dissolve in a full glass of water prior to intake; may use lemon juice for taste • Onset of action: 3–6 hrs
Polyethylene glycol (Miralax)	Init: 17 g daily MDD: 34 g PO daily	• Mix with 8 ounces of water, juice, coffee, or tea, • Onset of action: 24–96 hrs

Lubricant Laxatives—Penetrate and soften stool and interfere with reabsorption of water in the colon

Mineral oil (*Fleet Mineral Oil*)	*Init:* 45 mL PR as single dose MDD: 45 mL	• Avoid oral formulation due to risk of lipid pneumonitis. • Adverse effects: mild abdominal pain, fecal urgency, cramps • Onset of action: within 0.25 hr
Other Agents		
Linaclotide (*Linzess*)	*Init:* 145 mcg PO once daily MDD: 290 mcg	• Take on empty stomach at least 0.5 hr before the first meal of the day. • May cause diarrhea
Lubiprostone (*Amitiza*)	*Init:* 24 mcg PO twice daily MDD: 48 mcg	• Take with food and water. • May experience nausea, diarrhea, headache, abdominal pain, distention, flatulence
Methylnaltrexone (*Relistor*)	*Init:* Administered SC based on weight: <38 kg: 0.15 mg/kg/day 38 to <62 kg: 8 mg/day 62–114 kg: 12 mg/day	• For opioid-induced constipation • High cost of administration • Onset of action: 0.5–1 hr

MDD = maximum daily dose
From references 1, 9, 20, 23–30.

Table 3.5 Special Considerations for Constipation

Safe Prescribing	Complex Medication Use
• Individual bowel regimens are based on careful assessment and monitoring.	• Cost of medication versus pill burden should be considered and discussed.
• Assess for obstruction prior to initiating bowel stimulants.	• Estimated $800 million per year is spent on nonprescription laxatives.
• Use caution with over-the-counter medications because they may be contraindicated or duplicates of an already prescribed regimen.	• Improper use of enemas and suppositories may lead to bleeding, infection, electrolyte imbalance, and other adverse effects.

From references 7, 14, 35.

Pathophysiology

The pathophysiology of diarrhea is described by the specific cause or causes of increased stool water content and output. Potential causes are listed in Table 3.6 and include increased fluid secretion, decreased fluid absorption, or bowel hypermotility.[9,19]

Assessment

A careful history and assessment are crucial including the frequency, appearance, and number of stools and temporal correlation with medications, treatment, or meals. Secondary effects of diarrhea, such as fatigue, weakness, abdominal pain or cramping, dehydration, dizziness, weight loss, and skin breakdown, should also be identified. Constipation with a sudden onset of diarrhea is suspicious for fecal impaction or obstruction with overflow

Table 3.6 Pathophysiology of Diarrhea

Type	Causes
Increased fluid secretion (most difficult to control and often not preventable)	Inflammation
	Hormones
	Enterotoxins
	Chemotherapy, radiotherapy
Decreased fluid absorption	Medications (e.g., antibiotics)
	Hyperosmolar preparations/enteral feedings
	Laxative overuse
	Dietary: high-sorbitol diet, lactose intolerance
	Fistulas
Bowel hypermotility	Gastrointestinal malignancies
	Adhesions, fistulas
	Biliary/pancreatic or bowel obstructions
	Chemotherapy

From references 9, 19.

Box 3.3 Differential Diagnosis of Diarrhea

- Viral (e.g., noroviruses, rotaviruses)
- Bacterial (e.g., *Salmonella, Shigella, Escherichia coli, Listeria, Clostridium*)
- Protozoal (e.g., *Giardia lamblia, Cryptosporidium*)
- Medication (e.g., antibiotics, magnesium-containing agents, laxatives, chemotherapy)
- Inflammation (e.g., ulcerative colitis, Crohn's disease)
- Functional (e.g., irritable bowel syndrome, diverticulosis, anxiety)
- Malabsorption syndromes (e.g., sprue, pancreatic insufficiency, lactase deficiency)
- Treatment-related (e.g., post-gastrectomy dumping syndrome, fistulas)

From references 9, 12, 34.

---

diarrhea.[9,12] Medications should be reviewed for offending agents, such as laxatives, antibiotics, and chemotherapeutic agents.[8,19]

Signs of dehydration should be assessed. The physical examination focuses on the presence of oral candidiasis, hyperactive or hypoactive bowel sounds, abdominal distention, and tenderness. A rectal examination is performed if there is concern for fecal impaction.[12]

Additional testing may include stool specimen examination for pus, blood, fat, ova, or parasites as appropriate. Cultures and sensitivity testing can rule out opportunistic infections such as *Clostridium difficile* or other gastrointestinal infections.[9] An evaluation for electrolyte imbalance should be considered. If obstruction is suspected, an abdominal x-ray may be indicated[12] (Box 3.3).

Management

Initial management should focus on treatment of the underlying cause. Adequate hydration should be ensured and modification of medications or dietary factors should be considered.[33]

Pharmacologic Management

Identifying the cause of diarrhea guides pharmacotherapy. Treatment for specific causes of diarrhea includes pancreatic enzymes for steatorrhea or pancreatic insufficiency, cholestyramine for excess fecal bile acids or radiation-associated diarrhea, histamine antagonists for carcinoid syndrome, antibiotics, and mesalazine for ulcerative colitis.[12] Various nonspecific medications can be used for the general treatment of diarrhea and unless contraindicated, may help control the extent of symptoms (Tables 3.7, 3.8).

Management Interventional Techniques

For patients with limited mobility, fecal incontinence and persistent diarrhea in the acute care setting may warrant consideration of rectal catheter placement to divert stool away from both impaired and healthy skin. Patients on anticoagulation and antiplatelet therapy have an increased risk of gastrointestinal hemorrhage with rectal tubes and should be monitored closely.[41]

Table 3.7 Pharmacologic Management of Diarrhea

Generic name (*Brand name*)	Initial Dose (Init)	Comments
Bulk-forming agents—Absorb liquid in the gastrointestinal tract and increase the bulk consistency of stool		
Methylcellulose (*Citrucel*)	*Init:* 2 g 1–3 times daily as needed MDD: 6 g	Take with water to reduce risk of choking. Use caution in dehydrated patients. Onset of action: 24–48 hrs
Cholestyramine (*Questran*)	*Init:* 2–4 g 2–4 times daily MDD: 24 g	Bile acid-binding resin For chologenic diarrhea
Opioid agents—If cause of diarrhea is unknown and low suspicion for infection		
Codeine	*Init:* 10–60 mg PO 2–4 times daily MDD: Variable	Avoid use in diarrhea caused by poison or bacteria.
Diphenoxylate/Atropine (*Lomotil*)	*Init:* 5 mg/0.05 mg (2 tablets) PO, then 1 tablet (2.5 mg/0.025 mg) after each loose stool MDD: 20 mg	Avoid use in diarrhea caused by poison or bacteria. Onset of action: 0.75–1 hr
Loperamide (*Imodium*)	*Init:* 4 mg PO initially, followed by 2 mg after each unformed stool MDD: 16 mg	Avoid use in diarrhea caused by poison or bacteria.
Opium tincture	*Init:* 50 mg/5 mL 0.6 mL (range: 0.3–1 mL per dose) PO 4 times a day MDD: 6 mL	25 times stronger than paregoric or camphorated tincture of opium Monitor stools. Do not abruptly discontinue after prolonged use.
Camphorated tincture of opium (paregoric)	*Init:* 2 mg/5 mL 5–10 mL PO 1–4 times daily MDD: N/A	1/25 the strength of opium tincture Monitor stools. Do not abruptly discontinue after prolonged use.

Absorbants—Naturally occurring minerals that have adsorptive capacities		
Kaolin-pectin mixture (Kaopectate)	Init: 15–30 mL PO after each loose bowel movement	May decrease the absorption of drugs that chelate with aluminum
	MDD: 120 mL per 12 hrs	Onset of action: 24–48 hrs
Polycarbophil (Fiber-lax)	Init: 1,000 mg PO 1–4 times daily	Some products may contain calcium.
	MDD: 6,000 mg PO	Onset of action: 12–72 hrs
Salicylates—May have antisecretory, antimicrobial, and anti-inflammatory effects		
Bismuth subsalicylate (Pepto-Bismol)	Init: 524 mg PO every 30–60 minutes, as needed	For nonspecific acute diarrhea
	MDD: 4.2 g	Avoid in salicylate hypersensitivity.
		FDA approved for proctitis and ulcerative colitis
		May discolor stool
Somatostatin analogues—Inhibit diarrhea caused by hormone-secreting tumors of the pancreas and gastrointestinal tract		
Octreotide (Sandostatin)	Init: 300–600 mcg/day SC in 2–4 divided doses	May cause diarrhea, abdominal pain, nausea, and drowsiness
		High cost of administration
Other agents		
Ranitidine (Zantac)	Init: 150 mg twice daily	May be given with pancrelipase
	MDD: 300 mg	Reduces gastric acidity
Pancrelipase (Creon)	Init: Dose varies by brand	Individualize dose
		May be given with ranitidine or other H2 blocker
Vancomycin (Vancocin)	Init: 125 mg daily for 10 days	Diarrhea due to Clostridium difficile
Metronidazole (Flagyl)	Init: 400 mg 3 times daily for 10–14 days	Diarrhea due to Clostridium difficile
Cyproheptadine (Periactin)	Init: 4 mg 3 times daily	Carcinoid syndrome diarrhea

MDD = maximum daily dose
From references 25, 35–40.

Table 3.8 Special Considerations for Diarrhea

Safe-Prescribing	Complex Medication Use
• High-volume stool should not be masked with prescription or over-the-counter antidiarrheal agents.	• Cost of administration of treatment
• Severe diarrhea with rapid dehydration can lead to acute renal injury and, in extreme cases, shock. Further evaluation is imperative.	• Outpatient parenteral support may be necessary.
• Send stool specimen prior to suppressing output with medications.	• Cases of diarrhea accompanied by fever, nausea, vomiting, neutropenia, bleeding, or evidence of sepsis may require hospital admission.

From references 32, 33, 39.

Appropriate treatments should be consistent with the patient's goals of care and definition of quality of life.

Bowel Obstruction

Pathophysiology

Malignant bowel obstruction can occur at single or multiple levels and can be classified as mechanical or functional, partial or complete.[42]

Intra-abdominal tumors may be intraluminal or intramural. They can impair bowel function by occluding the lumen, causing intussusception, or by impairing peristalsis. Malignant adhesions can create multiple points of obstruction because they kink the bowel from an extramural site.[42,43] Duodenal obstruction is most related to cholangiocarcinoma and pancreatic malignancies, whereas distal obstruction is largely associated with primary colon and ovarian carcinomas.[42] In rare cases, obstruction is treatment-related from non-malignant adhesions following surgery or radiation.

Assessment

Duodenal obstruction presents with severe vomiting and emesis often containing undigested food. Pain or distention will often not be noted on examination. Obstructions of the small and large intestine both present with hyperactive bowel sounds with borborygmi. Nausea and vomiting will be more severe with obstruction higher along the gastrointestinal tract, whereas obstructions of the large intestine will produce delayed emesis with abdominal distention and colicky pain.[9, 42,44–46]

Radiologic imaging should be employed only if suspected findings can be treated. There tends to be an overreliance on abdominal x-rays, which are more cost-effective but less accurate than contrast radiographs.[42] Computed tomography (CT) scans remain the gold standard for diagnosis, with 94% accuracy in identifying the etiology of obstruction[9,44](Box 3.4).

Box 3.4 Differential Diagnosis of Malignant Bowel Obstruction

- Ileus
- Pseudo-obstruction
- Ogilvie syndrome
- Intra-abdominal sepsis

From references 9, 12.

Management

Symptoms associated with malignant bowel obstruction may be difficult to manage, such as nausea, vomiting, colic, and abdominal pains. Treatment should always be based on the patient's goals of care, symptom burden, and prognosis.[9,42,43,46]

Pharmacologic Management

The goal of pharmacologic management in obstruction is to provide symptomatic relief while minimizing the adverse effects of medications. Treatment includes analgesics, antisecretory drugs, glucocorticoids, and antiemetics; individualized treatment is encouraged.[47,48] Pharmacologic management options are listed in Table 3.9 and may be the sole treatment or used for symptom relief while anticipating surgical interventions.

For persistent pain, opioid analgesics are recommended; however, opioids tend to exacerbate colicky pain, and anticholinergic agents should be considered for pain relief.[47,49] Given the challenges with oral medications, parenteral, sublingual, and transdermal routes should be considered (Table 3.10).

Management Interventional Techniques

Multiple factors are associated with the selection of an intervention. Surgical intervention in advanced cancer is controversial and is determined by performance status, extent of disease, level of obstruction(s), presence of ascites, and goals of care.[44,45,56] Patients with progressive cancer despite tumor-directed therapy pose the greatest risk for surgeons.[42,45] In advanced cancer, often the risk of surgery outweighs any potential benefit, which may be difficult for patients and families to understand and accept.

Endoscopic procedures, such as gastric or colonic stenting, are a less invasive option and have been associated with quicker recovery in patients with a single focus of obstruction or locally advanced disease.[42] Stenting is contraindicated in patients with already established perforation or for rectal tumors because symptoms of tenesmus and incontinence may worsen.[42,57] Risks include stent migration and perforation.[44,56,57]

Management in patients with a poor prognosis, overt ascites, and carcinomatosis with multiple levels of obstruction is primarily supportive; placement of a venting gastrostomy tube can help to relieve symptoms. This may or may not allow the patient to tolerate some oral intake for pleasure, and it decreases pressure in the abdomen.[58]

Table 3.9 Pharmacologic Management of Obstruction

Generic name (Brand Name)	Initial Dose (Init)	Comments
Chlorpromazine (Thorazine)	Init: 10–25 mg q 4–6h as needed MDD: 1,000 mg	• To control nausea and vomiting • Sedating • Monitor for extrapyramidal symptoms (EPS). • Onset of action: 0.5–1 hr
Haloperidol (Haldol)	Init: 0.5–1 mg q 12h or q 4–6h as needed MDD: 100 mg PO	• To control nausea and vomiting • Monitor for EPS. • Onset of action: 0.5–1 hr
Metoclopramide (Reglan)	Init: 10 mg q 6–8h MDD: 60 mg PO; single dose not to exceed 20 mg	• Prokinetic; avoid in definitive or complete obstruction • May cause sedation, fatigue, and restlessness • Onset of action: 0.5–1 hr
Prochlorperazine (Compazine)	Init: 10 mg PO q 4–6h as needed or 25 mg PR q 6–12h as needed MDD: 50 mg/day PR; 40 mg/day PO or IM	• EPS, especially at high doses • Onset of action: 0.5–1 hr
Hyoscyamine (Levsin)	Init: 0.25–0.5 mg IV or SQ q 6h as needed or 0.125–0.25 mg PO or SL q 4h as needed MDD: 1.5 mg	• May cause blurred vision, confusion, constipation, dizziness, drowsiness, ileus, mydriasis, nausea/vomiting, nervousness, palpitations, sinus tachycardia, urinary retention/hesitancy, weakness • Onset of action: IV: 2–3 minutes; PO: 20–30 minutes
Octreotide (Sandostatin)	Init: 50–100 mcg IV/SQ q 8h MDD: Variable	• High cost of administration • May cause diarrhea, abdominal pain, flatulence, nausea, constipation • Onset of action: 0.5 hr
Scopolamine transdermal patch (Transderm Scop)	Init: 1.5 mg transdermal q 72h; 0.3–0.6 mg IV or SQ q 4h as needed MDD: 2.4 mg IV 1 transdermal patch q 72h	• May cause drowsiness or somnolence • Onset of action: transdermal, 4 hr; IV, 15–20 minutes
Dexamethasone (Decadron)	Init: 4 mg 1 or 2 times daily MDD: Variable	• Long-term use not recommended

From references 40, 47, 49, 50–53.

Table 3.10 Special Considerations for Malignant Bowel Obstruction

Safe Prescribing	Complex Medication Use
• Agents that promote gastrointestinal motility should be avoided with complete obstruction and used cautiously with partial obstruction.	• Combination regimens can improve quality of life but often require inpatient admissions due to cost and lack of availability in the community.
• Monitor patients on opioids and anticholinergics for side effects.	• Patient's goals of care should be reviewed.

From references 33, 39, 49, 50, 55.

Nasogastric tubes are often used as a temporary bridge to surgery and can be quite uncomfortable. These tubes provide short-term symptomatic relief in patients who do not qualify for a gastrostomy tube due to severe ascites or tumor infiltration of the stomach.[42,46]

Conclusion

Bowel symptoms do not occur in isolation and are often accompanied by decreased appetite, fatigue, and general malaise. Patients may experience loss of dignity that can lead to social isolation if not addressed. Crafting an individualized plan of care tailored to specific patient needs is an essential piece of quality care and promotes quality of life.

References

1. Candy B, Jones L, Goodman ML, Drake R, Tookman A. Laxatives or methylnaltrexone for the management of constipation in palliative care patients. *Cochrane Database Syst Rev.* 2011, Issue Art. No.: CD003448. doi: 10.1002/14651858.CD003448.pub3.

2. Clark K, Urban K, Currow DC. Current approaches to diagnosing and managing constipation in advanced cancer and palliative care. *J Palliat Med.* 2010; 13(4): 473–6.

3. Clark K, Currow DC. Constipation in palliative care: what do we use as definitions and outcome measures? *J Pain Symptom Manage.* 2013; 45(4): 753–62.

4. Strassels SA, Maxwell TL, Iyer S. Constipation in persons receiving hospice care. *J Pain Symptom Manage.* 2010; 40(6): 810–20.

5. Ishihara M, Iihara H, Okayasu S, et al. Pharmaceutical interventions facilitate premedication and prevent opioid-induced constipation and emesis in cancer patients. *Support Care Cancer.* 2010; 18: 1531–8.

6. Davis MP. Cancer constipation: are opioids really the culprit? *Support Care Cancer.* 2008; 16: 427–9.

7. Fabel PH, Shealy KIM. Diarrhea, constipation and irritable bowel syndrome. In: DiPiro JT, Talbert RL, et al., eds. *Pharmacotherapy: A Pathophysiologic Approach.* 9th ed. USA: McGraw-Hill Education; 2014:531–47.

8. American Gastroenterological Association. *Medical Position Statement on Constipation*. Available at http://www.gastrojournal.org/article/S0016-5085 (12)01545-4/fulltext#sec1. Accessed October 23, 2016.

9. Economou DC. Bowel management: constipation, diarrhea, obstruction, and ascites. In: Ferrell B, Coyle N, J Paice eds. *Oxford Textbook of Palliative Nursing*. 4th ed. New York: Oxford University Press; 2015:217–36.

10. Clark K, Smith JM, Currow DC. The prevalence of bowel problems reported in a palliative care population. *J Pain Symptom Manage*. 2012; 43(6): 993–1000.

11. Clemens KE, Faust M, Jaspers B, Mikus G. Pharmacological treatment of constipation in palliative care. *Curr Opin Support Palliat Carer*. 2013; 7(2): 183–91.

12. Sykes NP. Constipation and diarrhea. In: Walsh D, ed. *Palliative Medicine*. New York, NY: Saunders Elsevier; 2009:846–54.

13. Clark K, Lam LT, Agar M, Chye R, Currow DC. The impact of opioids, anticholinergic medications and disease progression on the prescription of laxatives in hospitalized patients: a retrospective analysis. *Palliat Med*. 2010; 24(4): 410–8.

14. McHugh ME, Miller-Saultz D. Assessment and management of gastrointestinal symptoms in advanced illness. *Prim Care Clin Office Pract*. 2011; 38: 225–46.

15. Agar M, Currow D, Plummer J, et al. Changes in anticholinergic load from regular prescribed medications in palliative care as death approaches. *Palliat Med*. 2009; 23: 257–65.

16. Librach SL, Bouvette M, De Angelis C, et al. Consensus recommendations for the management of constipation in patients with advanced, progressive illness. *J Pain Symptom Manage*. 2010; 40(5): 761–73.

17. Nagaviroj K, Chai Yong W, Fassbender K, Zhu G, Oneschuk D. Comparison of the constipation assessment scale and plain abdominal radiography in the assessment of constipation in advanced cancer patients. *J Pain Symptom Manage*. 2011; 42(2): 222–8.

18. McMillan SC, Williams FA. Validity and reliability of the constipation assessment scale. *Cancer Nurs*. 1989; 12(3): 183–8.

19. Richter JM. Approach to the patient with constipation. In: Goroll AH, Mulley AG, ed. *Primary Care Medicine*. 7th ed. Philadelphia, PA: Lippincott Williams & Wilkins; 2014:529–34.

20. Bharucha AE, Pemberton JH, Locke GR. 3rd American Gastroenterological Association technical review on constipation. *Gastroenterol*. 2013; 144: 218–38.

21. Clark K, Currow, DC. Assessing constipation in palliative care within a gastroenterology framework. *Palliat Med*. 2011; 26(6): 834–41.

22. Droney J, Ross J, Gretton S, et al. Constipation in cancer patients on morphine. *Support Care Cancer*. 2008; 16: 453–9.

23. Twycross R, Sykes N, Mihalyo M, Wilcock A. Stimulant laxatives and opioid-induced constipation. *J Pain Symptom Manage*. 2012; 43(2): 306–13.

24. Hurdon V, Viola R, Schroder C. How useful is docusate in patients at risk of constipation? A systematic review of the evidence in the chronically ill. *J Pain Symptom Manage*. 2000; 19: 130–6.

25. Gattuso JM, Kamm MA. Adverse effects of drugs used in the management of constipation and diarrhoea. *Drug Saf*. 1994; 10(1): 47–65.

26. Costilla VC, Foxx-Orenstein AE. Constipation: understanding mechanisms and management. *Clin Geriatr Med*. 2014; 30(1): 107–15.

27. Clausen MR, Mortensen PB. Lactulose, disaccharides and colonic flora. Clinical consequences. *Drugs*. 1997; 53: 930–42.

28. Agra Y, Sacristan A, Gonzalez M. Efficacy of senna versus lactulose in terminal cancer patients treated with opioids. *J Pain Symptom Manage*. 1998; 15: 1–7.

29. Wong BS, Camilleri M. Lubiprostone for the treatment of opioid-induced bowel dysfunction. *Expert Opin Pharmacother*. 2011; 12(6): 983–90.

30. Brick N. Laxatives or methylnaltrexone for the management of constipation in palliative care patients. *Clin J Oncol Nurs*. 2013; 17(1): 91–2.

31. Hjalte F, Berggren AC, Bergendahl H, Hjortsberg C. The direct and indirect costs of opioid-induced constipation. *J Pain Symptom Manage*. 2010; 40(5): 696–703.

32. Cherny NI. Evaluation and management of treatment-related diarrhea in patients with advanced cancer: a review. *J Pain Symptom Manage*. 2008; 36(4): 413–23.

33. von Gunten CF, Gafford E. Treatment of non-pain related symptoms. *Cancer J*. 2013; 19(5): 397–404.

34. Richter JM. Evaluation and management of diarrhea. In: Goroll AH, Mulley AG, ed. *Primary Care Medicine*. 7th ed. Philadelphia, PA: Lippincott Williams & Wilkins; 2014:517–28.

35. Phillips J. Kaopectate reformulation and upcoming labeling changes. *Drug Topics*. 2004; 148: 58.

36. Kent AJ, Banks MR. Pharmacological management of diarrhea. *Gastroenterol Clin North Am*. 2010; 39: 495–507.

37. Brunton LL, Chabner BA, Knollmann BC. *Goodman & Gilman's The Pharmacological Basis of Therapeutics*, 12th ed. New York, NY: McGraw-Hill; 2011.

38. Prommer E. Role of codeine in palliative care. *J Opioid Manage*. 2011; 7(5): 401–6.

39. Craig DS. Constipation and diarrhea. In: Strickland JM, ed. *Palliative Pharmacy Care*. USA: American Society of Health-System Pharmacists, Inc.; 2009:115–25.

40. Mercadente S. The role of octreotide in palliative care. *J Pain Symptom Manage*. 1994; 9(6): 406–11.

41. Mulhall AM, Jindal SK. Massive gastrointestinal hemorrhage as a complication of the Flexi-Seal fecal management system. *Am J Crit Care*. 2013; 22(6): 537–43.

42. Soriano A, Davis MP. Malignant bowel obstruction: individualized treatment near the end of life. *Cleveland Clinic J Med*. 2011; 78(3): 197–206.

43. Wright FC, Chakraborty A, Helyer L, Moravan V, Selby D. Predictors of survival in patients with non-curative stage IV cancer and malignant bowel obstruction. *J Surg Oncol*. 2010; 101: 425–9.

44. Laval G, Marcelin-Benazech B, Guirimand F, et al. Recommendations for bowel obstructions with peritoneal carcinomatosis. *J Pain Symptom Manage*. 2014; 48(1): 75–91.

45. Olson TJP, Pinkerton C, Brasel KJ, Scwarze ML. Palliative surgery for malignant bowel obstruction from carcinomatosis. *JAMA Surg*. 2014; 149(4): 383–92.

46. Lynch M, Dahlin C, Bakitas M. Bowel obstruction and delirium: managing difficult symptoms at the end of life. *Clin J Oncol Nurs*. 2011; 16(4): 391–8.

47. Ripamonti, C. Twycross R, Baines M, et al. Clinical-practice recommendations for the management of bowel obstruction in patients with end-stage cancer. *Supportive Care Cancer.* 2001; 9: 223–33.

48. Sykes N. Constipation and diarrhea. In: Hanks G, Cherny NI, Christakis NA, et al., eds. *Oxford Textbook of Palliative Medicine.* 4th ed. Oxford: Oxford University Press; 2010:833–50.

49. Ripamonti C, Mercadente S, Groff L, et al. Role of octreotide, scopolamine butylbromide, and hydration in symptom control of patients with inoperable bowel obstruction and nasogastric tubes: a prospective randomized trial. *J Pain Symptom Manage.* 2000; 19: 23–34.

50. Ripamonti C, Mercadente S. Pathophysiology and management of malignant bowel obstruction. In: Hanks G, Cherny NI, Christakis NA, et al., eds. *Oxford Textbook of Palliative Medicine.* 4th ed. Oxford, UK: Oxford University Press; 2010:850–63.

51. Laval, G. Girardier J, Lassauniere JM, et al. The use of steroids in the management of inoperable intestinal obstruction in terminal cancer patients: do they remove the obstruction? *Palliat Med.* 2000; 14: 3–10.

52. Tuca A, Guell E, Martinez-Losada E, Codorniu N. Malignant bowel obstruction in advanced cancer patients: epidemiology, management, and factors influencing spontaneous resolution. *Cancer Manag Res.* 2012; 4: 159–69.

53. Laval G, Rousselot H, Toussaint-Martel S, et al. SALTO: a randomized, multi-center study assessing octreotide LAR in inoperable bowel obstruction. *Bull Cancer.* 2012; 99: E1–E9.

54. Ripamonti C, Easson AM, Gerdes H. Management of malignant bowel obstruction. *Eur J Cancer.* 2008; 44(8): 1105–15.

55. Marukami H, Matsumoto H, Nakamura M, Hirai T, Yamaguchi Y. Octreotide acetate-steroid combination therapy for malignant gastrointestinal obstruction. *Anticancer Res.* 2013; 33: 5557–60.

56. Abbott S, Eglinton TW, Ma Y, et al. Predictors of outcome in palliative colonic stent placement for malignant obstruction. *Br J Surg.* 2014; 101: 121–6.

57. Alford T, Ghosh S, Wong C, Schiller D. Clinical outcomes of stenting for colorectal obstruction at a tertiary centre. *J Gastrointest Canc.* 2014; 45: 61–5.

58. Mori M, Bruera E, Dev R. Complications of a gastrostomy tube used for decompression of an inoperable bowel obstruction in a patient with advanced cancer. *J Pain Symptom Manage.* 2009; 38(3): 466–72.

Chapter 4

Challenging Symptoms: Dry Mouth, Hiccups, Fevers, Pruritus, and Sleep Disorders

Barton T. Bobb and Devon Fletcher

Key Points
• Fever may require scheduled antipyretic treatment at end-of-life if it is believed to be distressing. • Dry mouth is a common symptom among palliative care patients, especially cancer patients. • Pruritus can be challenging to treat; determining the cause when possible can help tailor treatment.

Pruritus

Pruritus is often associated with pathological or chronic itch causing a desire to scratch. This scratch reflex is meant to be a protective mechanism, but when this sensation becomes chronic, there can be resulting emotional and physical consequences.[1] Pruritus is a frequently underreported symptom.[2] However, the impact on quality of life, sleep, anxiety, and depression can be very distressing.

The physiology of the itch sensation transmission is not well understood. It was initially thought to be a subset of the pain transmission pathway but is now believed to be transmitted from the peripheral nervous system by slow, unmyelinated type C nerve fibers to the central nervous system (CNS), distinct from the type C polymodal fibers that carry aching, dull, or burning pain sensations.[1,3–5]

Etiology

Finding the source of the itching can be challenging, but determining the cause may help direct the choice of treatment. The direct cause cannot always be determined, or patients may have overlapping or multiple causes of pruritus.[6,7]

Primary Dermatologic Causes

Pruritus is the most commonly reported symptom in dermatologic disorders as a whole.[2] Often, itch-producing stimuli are short-lived or self-limiting and, if needed, can be treated effectively by a primary care provider or other first-line providers. Causes of primary dermatologic conditions can range from dry skin and insect bites to dermatologic malignancies.

Systemic Diseases

Pruritus can manifest in many systemic diseases (Table 4.1). Approximately 70% of patients with cholestatic liver disease from various causes reported pruritus.[3,8,9] Bilirubin accumulation is thought to be the underlying cause, but how this causes itching is largely unknown.[10–13] Chronic renal insufficiency is another systemic disease with a high symptom burden from pruritus, especially in patients on chronic hemodialysis.[2,14] Metabolic derangements in renal disease such as hypercalcemia, hyperphosphatemia, and hypermagnesemia seem to contribute independently to pruritus as well.[15] Endocrinopathies

Table 4.1 Systemic Causes of Pruritus

Biliary and hepatic disease
Chronic renal insufficiency/uremia
Endocrinopathy
Hyper/hypothyroid
Hyperparathyroid
Diabetes mellitus
Carcinoid syndrome
Infectious diseases
HIV/AIDS
Infectious hepatitis
Parasitic disease
Prion disease
Hematologic/oncologic
Lymphoma/leukemia
Systemic mastocytosis
Multiple myeloma
Polycythemia vera
Iron deficiency anemia
Autoimmune
Dermatitis herpetiformis
Dermatomyositis
Linear immunoglobulin A
Medications
Opioids
Amphetamines
Cocaine
Niacin
Aspirin

such as hyperparathyroidism, both hypothyroidism and hyperthyroidism, and diabetes are all associated with itching.[1,2,16,17] Multiple hematopoietic disorders, ranging from more benign iron deficiency anemia to malignancies such as lymphoma and multiple myeloma, can cause itching or chronic pruritus. T-cell lymphomas, in particular Sézary syndrome, are characterized by a high incidence of pruritus and commonly require the assistance of a palliative provider for more advanced interventions.[18,19] Infectious diseases can cause various local and systemic pruritus. There has been an increasing recognition of chronic pruritus seen in HIV-positive patients; it appears to be independent of the incidence of primary dermatologic sources of itch.[20,21]

Medications

Any medication can cause itching from an allergic reaction or sensitivity. Certain medications or illicit drugs commonly known to cause itching include opiates, amphetamines, cocaine, niacin, and aspirin.[1,2]

Neurologic

Patients with stroke or brain tumor (either primary or due to metastatic disease) can have a centrally mediated itch. There are also peripheral neuropathic itch syndromes, such as post-herpetic itch and notalgia paresthetica.[1,7,22]

Psychiatric

Pruritus is reported to be common in psychiatric conditions, such as psychosis or delirium, but epidemiologic data on the actual prevalence are lacking.[2] In addition to causing pruritus, anxiety and depression are thought to worsen the patient's ability to cope with pruritus of other etiologies.[23]

Treatment

Treatment of systemic pruritus is often difficult. Particularly frustrating is that the mainstays of treatment for primary dermatologic pruritus are often not helpful for systemic causes. If the pruritus is from a disease process or medication that cannot be removed, then treatment modalities range from topical therapies to systemic medications or invasive interventions in which the symptom burden should outweigh the risk of the treatment.

Initial nonpharmacologic interventions include patient and family education on methods to decrease itching, such as wearing light clothing and lowering the room temperature. The APRN should also continue to monitor the patient's skin for excoriation and secondary infections from scratching.[24]

Topical Treatments

Topical ointments and barrier creams are always available and should be used (Box 4.1). However, they are less likely to be helpful when pruritus is due to a systemic cause, which is the more likely type to be seen within palliative care.[25,26]

Systemic Treatments

Systemic therapies are varied (Table 4.2). When possible, therapy should be directed toward the source of pruritus. Antihistamines are particularly helpful for pruritus that is known to be histamine-mediated. They are generally trialed for all types of pruritus at some point because they have a relatively

Box 4.1 Topical Treatments of Pruritus
Calamine
Menthol
Oatmeal bath
Antihistamines
Steroids
Capsaicin

benign side-effect profile. Side effects commonly include drowsiness and dry mouth; the former can actually be helpful if the patient is experiencing pruritus at night affecting sleep, but can limit use if causing sedation during the day.[25]

Opiate rotation should be considered for patients experiencing pruritus associated with opiate use. If this is not possible, the use of an opioid receptor antagonist such as naloxone or naltrexone may be helpful. Intravenous naloxone is not a realistic treatment option for outpatient or home management or for long-term use. Its half-life is too short, but it can be given by intravenous infusion for acute symptoms.[27,28] Opiate antagonism can produce side effects similar to opiate withdrawal, and patients should be warned of this prior to use.

Table 4.2 Common Systemic Treatments of Pruritus
Antihistamines
Diphenhydramine (PO, IV)
Doxylamine (PO)
Hydroxyzine (PO, IM)
Rifampicin (PO)
Sequestrants
Cholestyramine (PO)
Colestipol (PO)
Opioid Receptor Antagonists
Naloxone (IV)
Naltrexone (PO, IM)
Neuroleptics
Gabapentin (PO)
Pregabalin (PO)
Antidepressants
SSRIs (PO)
Mirtazapine (PO)
Doxepin (PO)
Antiemetics
Ondansetron (PO, IV)
Aprepitant (PO)

Sequestrant medications, such as cholestyramine and colestipol, are often used on a first-line basis to control pruritus in cholestatic liver disease.[1,28,29] Compliance difficulties can arise because these medications can be unpleasant to swallow, and there should be a 4-hour interval before taking other oral medications.[28]

Rifampicin has been found to be helpful for pruritus in hepatic cholestasis as a second-line agent. Liver biochemistries should be checked periodically because the antibiotic may cause toxic hepatitis in about 15% of cases, and patients should be counseled about the signs of liver failure.[1,28,29]

Neuroleptics like gabapentin seem to be effective for neurologic causes of itching.[1,28] Both gabapentin and pregabalin are showing promise for the treatment of pruritus associated with uremia.[28,30] Serotonin reuptake inhibitors, such as sertraline, paroxetine, and fluvoxamine,[1,7,28] as well as mirtazapine, a tetracyclic antidepressant, and doxepin, a tricyclic antidepressant, have all shown some benefit in pruritus caused by various etiologies.[1,7,25,28]

Antiemetics, such as ondansetron, a type 3 (5-HT$_3$) serotonin receptor antagonist, may relieve some types of pruritus. Further randomized controlled trials suggest antiemetics may not be helpful for pruritus related to hepatic cholestatic disease and chronic renal disease.[1,7,25,31] Aprepitant, a neurokinin receptor-1 (NKR 1) antagonist used as an antiemetic, blocks the binding of substance P and has been particularly helpful in patients with T-cell lymphoma.[7,18,25]

Agents that are less commonly used to treat pruritus include immunosuppressants,[25] tranquilizers, sedatives, and heparin.[28] Topical steroids are frequently used for dermatologic disorders, but oral steroids are thought to help reduce itch only if an inflammatory component is present. Because of the side effects of long-term steroid use, providers should exhaust other treatments before using steroids for systemic pruritus.[25]

Interventional Treatments
Several interventions for pruritus (mostly pruritus caused by liver disease) have been developed for patients with symptoms refractory to less invasive treatments (Box 4.2). Prognosis and ability to withstand these interventions would depend on overall clinical status. Patients with primary biliary cirrhosis with cholestatic disease may be liver transplant candidates based on their

Box 4.2 Interventional Treatments for Pruritus

Acupuncture
Biliary drainage
Hemodialysis
Liver transplantation
Parathyroidectomy
Phototherapy
Plasmapheresis
Transcutaneous nerve stimulation

pruritus symptoms alone.[13] Extracorporeal albumin dialysis[29,32] and biliary drainage have also been shown to relieve intractable pruritus in primary biliary cirrhosis.[27] Additional investigation needs to be performed, but initial observations seem to suggest that phototherapy[1,25,28] and plasmapheresis[25–27] may be beneficial in relieving chronic pruritus as well. Therapies such as acupuncture and transcutaneous nerve stimulation may also be worth exploring.[1]

Hiccups

Hiccups represent an involuntary spasm of the diaphragm and accessory respiratory muscles. The causes of hiccups can be varied, but they generally result from an irritation of the diaphragm directly or of the nervous system controlling this muscle. The hiccup reflex involves: the afferent vagal, phrenic, and sympathetic nerves; the brainstem; and the efferent phrenic nerve to the diaphragm. Gastric distention and gastroesophageal reflux are among the more common causes of persistent hiccups. Toxicity, as in infections or uremia, and CNS or direct phrenic nerve irritation are also potential causes of hiccups.[32,33–38] Awareness that medications such as corticosteroids have been linked to hiccups may be beneficial for palliative APRNs working with oncology patients.[39,40]

Attempting vagal maneuvers, nasopharyngeal stimulation, and inducing hypercapnia with hyperventilation are among the initial physical interventions that may be successful.[32,40] If symptoms persist or recur at a frequency where the benefit of interventions outweighs the potential side effects, several medications have been tried with some success, although, as mentioned, limited data exist for these treatments. Chlorpromazine, a phenothiazine first-generation antipsychotic, is the only medication approved by the US Food and Drug Administration (FDA) for the treatment of persistent hiccups.[32,38] Doses of oral chlorpromazine for hiccups are typically lower than those for antipsychotic effects. Side effects include dizziness, drowsiness, dystonia, neuroleptic malignant syndrome, and tardive dyskinesia. These side effects can limit the ability to use this medication as a first-line therapy.[38]

Metoclopramide, a prokinetic agent with dopamine receptor antagonist properties, may also be of benefit for hiccups.[41,42] If hiccups are due to gastric distention, this may be a particularly beneficial therapeutic agent to resolve the underlying cause of the hiccups. Side effects include drowsiness, agitation, tardive dyskinesia, dizziness, and confusion, which may limit use. QTc prolongation may occur, and monitoring may be indicated.

Haloperidol, specifically via the intramuscular route, was supported in older literature as a treatment for intractable hiccups based on several case reports,[43] but no new data confirms this. Baclofen, a gamma-aminobutyric acid (GABA) analog used as a muscle relaxant, is emerging as a promising treatment for intractable hiccups.[32,44-47] Further evaluation of this treatment in the palliative patient population is needed, however, because most data are specific to neurological conditions. Baclofen's potential side effects include respiratory depression, sedation, and asthenia but are most common in patients with impaired renal function,[46] and, overall, some data suggest that this therapy has minimal adverse events.[44,47]

Gabapentin has also been identified as a potential low-burden second-line therapy for intractable hiccups, including in advanced cancer patients.[32,38,48,49] Drowsiness is identified as the major potential side effect, but it is otherwise well tolerated.[49]

Antihypertensive medications, such as nifedipine,[50] a calcium channel blocker, and carvedilol,[51] a beta-blocker, have significantly fewer data supporting their use for hiccups. If side effects from more established treatments limit use, these may be alternative therapies if the patient's blood pressure levels support their use. Various other medications, such as benzodiazepines, methylphenidate, serotonergic agonists,[32,33] olanzapine, valproic acid, cisapride, omeprazole,[45,48] lidocaine,[32,52] amitriptyline, ketamine, and amantadine[53] all have limited case reports or case series supporting their use.

Therapeutic interventions, such as surgical or radiofrequency nerve ablation,[32,54] diaphragmatic pacing,[32] and alternative therapies such as acupuncture[32,55,56] have shown effectiveness. However, further studies are needed.

Various nonpharmacologic, pharmacologic, and alternative therapies, including invasive interventions, may be beneficial for this relatively rare symptom.[32,34,48,49]

Dry Mouth

Dry mouth, or xerostomia, is common in cancer patients and patients at the end of life.[57–59] The differential diagnosis can be divided into four areas: decreased saliva secretion, dehydration, erosion of the buccal mucosa, and miscellaneous.[58,59]

Saliva secretion is regulated by both sympathetic and parasympathetic processes and involves a number of different pathways, so the pathophysiology of hyposalivation can be traced to several potential causes, including a slight disruption of the muscarinic receptors to outright obliteration of parenchymal tissue.[60] The parotid, submandibular, and sublingual glands work together to produce saliva and maintain proper consistency, so damage to any of them will affect not only the amount but also the viscosity of the saliva.[59]

Decreased saliva secretion can be caused by radiation to the head and neck, chemotherapy, a variety of medications (e.g., anticholinergics, antihistamines, tricyclic antidepressants, opioids, and sedatives), and some medical conditions (e.g., autoimmune disorders, infections, and sarcoidosis).[58,59]

Erosion of the buccal mucosa can also be caused by a variety of medical conditions (e.g., HIV/AIDS, Sjögren syndrome, systemic lupus erythematosus, and diabetes mellitus) plus chemotherapy and radiation, where higher doses and more radiation treatments also directly affect the extent and length of impairment in saliva production.[58,59] Xerostomia from dehydration can occur as a result of vomiting, diarrhea, dysphagia, oxygen use, and fever, whereas mental health issues, such as depression or anxiety, are potential miscellaneous causes of xerostomia.[59,60]

A basic clinical history and focused exam should be sufficient to make the diagnosis and determine the likely etiology.[57] The inside of the mouth can be examined for signs of xerostomia, such as dry mucosa and tongue,

Table 4.3 Pharmacologic Xerostomia Treatments

Saliva Stimulants	Saliva Substitutes
Pilocarpine 5–10 mg tid (primarily muscarinic agonist)	Mucin-based (e.g., Saliva Orthana)
Cevimeline 15–30 mg tid (muscarinic)	Carboxymethyl-cellulose-based (e.g., BioXtra)
From references 57, 59, 61.	

and ulceration. Two simple bedside tests to evaluate for xerostomia are: the cracker test, in which the patient is diagnosed to have xerostomia if unable to eat a cracker without drinking something; and the tongue depressor test, which diagnoses xerostomia if the tongue depressor sticks to the tongue after placement.[59] There are also certain assessment tools, such as the University of Michigan Xerostomia tool, that allow patients to rate their symptoms.[59]

The management of xerostomia relies on potentially complex medication use as well as nonpharmacologic interventions (Table 4.3, Box 4.3). A general approach to management involves treating any underlying conditions (e.g., candidiasis), reviewing medications and changing those that may be contributing to xerostomia, finding ways to stimulate salivation, using saliva substitutes to replace lost saliva, and managing the xerostomia holistically in general.[59]

Mucin-based saliva substitutes appear to be better tolerated than carboxymethyl-cellulose-based ones, and sprays overall better than gels.[57,59] Contraindications to taking pilocarpine include asthma, bronchitis/chronic obstructive pulmonary disease, glaucoma, and heart, kidney, or liver disease.[57,59] Cevimeline should not be used in patients with acute iritis, uncontrolled asthma, or narrow-angle glaucoma.[57]

Preventative oral care interventions for patients with xerostomia should be encouraged. This includes regular teeth brushing with fluoridated toothpaste, water rinse containing ½ teaspoon baking soda in a cup of water, and use of a daily antimicrobial rinse.[60] Oral care is especially important throughout the disease course, including at end of life for continued comfort.[59]

Potential interventional techniques to treat xerostomia are acupuncture and intraductal gene therapy. Acupuncture is inserted via the parotid gland, but does not have sufficient evidence to recommend it. Gene therapy is in its early stages of research.[61]

Box 4.3 Nonpharmacologic Xerostomia Treatments

Sugar-free chewing gum

Organic acids (ascorbic acid, citric acid, malic acid)

Water/peppermint water

Electrostimulation (embedded in a custom-made mouthguard)

Diet modifications (e.g., soft foods, increased fluid intake with meals, avoiding sugary and spicy foods)

From references 57, 59, 61.

Fevers

Fever is generally defined as a rise in oral body temperature above 38°C (100.4°F).[24] The pathophysiology of fever is based on the presence of pyrogens, substances that produce fever, inducing the hypothalamus to reset the body temperature set point.[62] Pathogens release exogenous pyrogens, and the destruction of pathogens causes the body to produce endogenous pyrogens, namely interleukin-1 and -6, interferons, and tumor necrosis factor, but both types of pyrogens can ultimately induce fever.[62]

Clinically, fever often presents in three stages: chill, fever, and flush.[24] During the chill phase, the body is reacting to its new temperature set point. The body generates heat through shivering and tries to prevent heat loss through vasoconstriction.[24] During the fever phase, the body raises its temperature to meet the new set point, resulting in a warm feeling, lethargy, and possible dehydration or even seizures. In the flush stage, the body tries to acclimate to the new set point through diaphoresis and vasodilation.[24] Certain populations, such as immunocompromised patients, older adults, newborns, and those taking steroids, may not mount a fever response with an infection.[63]

The assessment of patients with fever usually begins with a detailed history and exam. The extent of evaluation and further workup may vary greatly depending on the patient's prognosis and established goals.[63] Some of the most common differential diagnoses of fever in palliative care patients include infection (the most common etiology), medications, paraneoplastic-related fevers, neurologic damage, and inflammation.[62] Neutropenic patients are particularly susceptible to infections; some common sources include wounds, the bloodstream and urinary tract, implanted vascular access devices, pneumonia, and the gastrointestinal tract.[62]

If a workup is pursued and the source of the fever is identified, treatment of the underlying condition may involve both interventional techniques (e.g., drainage of an abscess) and complex medication options (e.g., intravenous antibiotics). In some instances, empiric antibiotics could be initiated without further workup. This may be appropriate when patients have a colonized infection and antibiotics curb the infection just enough to ward off fevers.

However, when patients are actively dying, even empiric antibiotics are usually no longer indicated.[24] In fact, even symptomatic treatment of fever is not always necessary or appropriate. Fevers may not cause discomfort, but breaking the fever—and the likely resulting sweats—could cause discomfort.[62] There is also some indication that low-level fevers can have a protective function. It is ultimately the patient's (or the family's if the patient cannot communicate) decision whether the fever is bothering him or her.[62]

For symptomatic treatment of fever, the major medication options include acetaminophen 325 to 650 mg q 4–6h (orally, intravenously, or rectally), non-steroidal anti-inflammatory drugs (e.g., naproxen 225–500 mg orally q 12h, intravenous ketorolac 15–30 mg q 6h, ibuprofen 200–400 mg orally q 4–6h, or indomethacin 50 mg orally or rectally q 8h), or aspirin 325 to 650 mg orally or rectally q 6h plus corticosteroids.[62] Generally speaking, antipyretics' action centers on preventing the production of prostaglandin E2.[63] When antipyretics are administered for symptomatic relief, it is best to schedule them around the clock to avoid fluctuations in body temperature and diaphoresis with fever.[24]

Nonpharmacologic interventions to treat fevers need to be chosen carefully. Many of the treatments historically used to bring down fevers, such as ice packs, cooling blankets, cold sponge baths, or a fan blowing directly on the patient, can cause more discomfort by making the patient too cold and inducing shivering.[24] Instead, some measures that can be safely implemented to help maintain patient comfort include keeping the room temperature at a comfortable level, ensuring that the patient's bed linen and clothing are clean and dry, offering cool liquids to drink for those who can drink, and ensuring that the patient's lips are kept moist.[24,62]

Cool, not cold, cloths may help, as well as light bedding. Mouth care should be continued since fever causes dry mouth.[24] Patients and family members may need ongoing support and reassurance when the decision is made not to treat the underlying cause of a fever or its symptoms. This is particularly true if the fever does not appear to be causing discomfort to the dying patient. However, if family members insist that their loved one receive symptomatic fever treatment, it may be an appropriate and palliative measure to do so.[62] When patients require symptomatic treatment for fevers earlier in the course of their disease, patients and families may require extensive education and reminders about the potential dangers of excessive nonsteroidal anti-inflammatory drugs or acetaminophen use.

Sleep Disorders

Sleep disorders and their associated insomnia or lack of quality sleep are a potentially very disturbing issue for palliative patients. Broadly speaking, the American Academy of Sleep Medicine classifies sleep disorders into four categories: disorders of extreme somnolence; disorders of the sleep–wake cycle; difficulty initiating or maintaining sleep; and dysfunction of sleep, sleep stages, or incomplete arousal.[64] A workup to differentiate primary insomnia from another specific sleep disorder may include the Epworth Sleepiness Scale questionnaire, an overnight polysomnogram followed by daytime multiple sleep latency testing if evaluating for narcolepsy, use of an actigraph to study sleep–wake patterns, and other miscellaneous tests.[66] A polysomnogram positive for sleep apnea would likely be followed by a trial of continuous positive airway pressure (CPAP), possibly even done halfway through the night of a polysomnogram if the results are blatantly positive. A survey of 76 palliative care clinic patients indicated that about 40% met criteria for restless leg syndrome that reduced their quality of life[67] (Box 4.4).

The most common sleep disorder is some form of simple/primary insomnia (occurs in 23–61% of cancer patients), which is the focus of the remainder of this section.[64] The normal architecture of sleep involves two major phases: rapid and non-rapid eye movement sleep (REM and NREM).[64] During REM sleep, sometimes also called "dream sleep," the brain is very active, whereas NREM sleep consists of four increasingly deep, quiet, and restorative periods of sleep that together make up one sleep cycle of approximately

Box 4.4 Differential Diagnosis of Major Sleep Disorders

Primary insomnia

Sleep apnea

Restless leg syndrome

Narcolepsy

Parasomnia

From reference 65.

90 minutes.[64] The pathophysiology of insomnia is potentially quite complex because it involves an increased level of arousal of the brain, including higher activity during NREM sleep. Genetic factors may predispose individuals to be more sensitive to external factors, such as caffeine or stress, that can subsequently disrupt the sleep–wake cycle.[64] Some other biological differences found in patients with chronic insomnia include higher levels of adrenocorticotropic hormone (ACTH), cortisol, and adrenaline release and increased body temperature compared to patients who sleep normally.[64]

The assessment of insomnia begins by obtaining a thorough sleep history from the patient and any sleeping partner. It involves an evaluation of sleep chronology, environment, and hygiene in addition to any physical symptoms, medical conditions, and spiritual concerns.[65] The sleep assessment questionnaires that have been used most frequently in research include the Epworth Sleepiness Scale, the Insomnia Severity Index, and the Pittsburgh Sleep Quality Index; the Insomnia Severity Index appears to have the most consistency and reliability regarding cancer patients in particular.[68]

A review of generally accepted sleep hygiene behaviors may help: (1) a regular sleep time and wakeup time, (2) use of the bed only for sleep and sexual activity, (3) avoidance of lying in bed awake for more than about 30 minutes if unable to fall asleep at scheduled sleep time, (4) return to bed only when sleepy, (5) the use of naps, (6) reduction of dietary caffiene intake in food or beverages, (7) activity level monitoring, and (8) sleep environment evaluation.

By assessing the sleep chronology, determination of the course of the patient's insomnia can be more clearly related to sleep onset, maintenance, or both.[65] If the insomnia is an ongoing problem, there may often be a medical, psychological, or neurological disorder that is at least partially responsible.[65] Medications may cause frequent awakening throughout the night, and early morning awakening is often related to depression.[65]

Medical conditions can also contribute to insomnia, including worsening of a chronic problem, such as chronic obstructive pulmonary disease or congestive heart failure, a recent or deepening depression that may also be accompanied by anxiety, a variety of medications to treat such conditions (e.g., corticosteroids, stimulants), or previously mentioned sleep disorders like restless leg syndrome.[65] Physical symptoms such as pain, shortness of breath, or cough may interfere with sleep initiation or maintenance. Spiritual distress associated with the fear of dying while asleep, together with other anxiety and fear of uncertainty, may precipitate reluctance to fall asleep and nightmares.[65] The only sleep disorder that routinely uses an interventional technique for management is obstructive sleep apnea, which may be treated with use of a continuous positive airway pressure (CPAP) machine at night or, in some cases, can improve with uvulopalatopharyngoplasty surgery.

The management of insomnia generally consists of complex medication management and nonpharmacologic interventions. The major classes of medications approved by the FDA to treat insomnia are benzodiazepines, benzodiazepine receptor agonists, non-benzodiazepine receptor agonists, and melatonin-receptor agonists.[64] Some of the other major classes of drugs frequently used to treat insomnia include antidepressants, atypical antipsychotics, and antihistamines.[69]

Benzodiazepine and non-benzodiazepine agonists both act on the GABA receptor complex. The APRN should use caution if a patient already taking opioids is given benzodiazepines. For some patients, a synergistic effect may occur, and more sedation may ensue. Non-benzodiazepine agonists do not affect the sleep architecture and tend to have fewer side effects, especially longer-lasting ones (e.g., less risk for abuse, dependence, and lingering oversedation).[64] Melatonin-receptor agonists act on MT_1 and MT_2 receptors, are believed to be involved in normal sleep–wake cycle regulation, and have fewer side effects and no risk for abuse or dependence; only ramelteon has FDA approval.[64] The other classes of drugs are used due to their sedating properties[64,69] (Table 4.4).

Table 4.4 Pharmacologic Options to Manage Insomnia

Medication and Dosage	Major Side Effects
Benzodiazepine Receptor Agonists	
Temazepam 7.5–15 mg	Drowsiness, confusion
Triazolam 0.125 mg	Amnesia, drowsiness
Lorazepam 0.5–4 mg	Respiratory depression, sedation
Non-benzodiazepine Receptor Agonists	
Zolpidem 5–10 mg (IR), Zolpidem 6.25–12.5 mg (ER)	Sedation, dizziness
Eszopiclone 1–3 mg	Headache, drowsiness, dizziness
Antidepressants	
Trazodone 25–100 mg	Sedation, confusion, headache
Mirtazapine 15–30 mg	Constipation, sedation, xerostomia
Melatonin-Receptor Agonist	
Ramelteon 8 mg	CNS depression, headache
Atypical Antipsychotics	
Olanzapine 5–10 mg	Extrapyramidal side effects, drowsiness
Antihistamines	
Diphenhydramine 25–50 mg	Dizziness, headache, sedation
Doxylamine 25 mg	Paradoxical CNS arousal, dizziness, sedation

From references 64, 66, 69.

References

1. Pittelkow MR, Loprinzi CL. Pruritus and sweating in palliative medicine. In: Hanks G, Cherny NI, Christakis NA, Fallon M, Kaasa S, Portenoy RK, eds. *Oxford Textbook of Palliative Medicine*. 4th ed. New York, NY: Oxford University Press; 2011:934–51.

2. Weisshaar E, Matterne U. Epidemiology of itch. Chapter 2 in: Carstens E, Akiyama T, eds. Itch: Mechanisms and Treatment. Boca Raton, FL: CRC Press; 2014. Available at https://www.ncbi.nlm.nih.gov/books/NBK200924/. Accessed October 24, 2016.

3. Han L, Dong X. Itch mechanisms and circuits. *Annu Rev Biophys*. 2014; 43: 331–55.

4. Ringkamp M, Schepers RJ, Shimada SG, et al. A role for nociceptive, myelinated nerve fibers in itch sensation. *J Neurosci*. 2011; 31: 14841–9.

5. Kuraishi Y. Recent advances in the study of itching: potential new therapeutic targets for pathological pruritus. *Biol Pharm Bull*. 2013; 36 (8): 1228–34.

6. Reamy B, Bunt C, Fletcher S, Bergguist E. A diagnostic approach to pruritus. *Am Fam Physician*. 2011; 84(2): 195–202.

7. Kfoury LW, Jurdi MA. Uremic pruritus. *J Nephrol*. 2012; 25: 644–52.

8. Bunchorntavakul C, Reddy KR. Pruritus in chronic cholestatic liver disease. *Clin Liver Dis*. 2012; 16: 331–46.

9. Oude Elferink RP, Kremer AE, Martens JJ, Beuers UH. The molecular mechanism of cholestatic pruritus. *Dig Dis*. 2011; 29(1): 66–71.

10. Alemi F, Kwon E, Poole DP, et al. The TGR5 receptor mediates bile acid–induced itch and analgesia. *J Clin Investig*. 2013; 123: 1513–30.

11. Kremer AE, Martens JJ, Kulik W, et al. Lysophosphatidic acid is a potential mediator of cholestatic pruritus. *Gastroenterol*. 2010; 139: 1008–18.

12. European Association for the Study of the Liver. EASL Clinical Practice Guidelines: management of cholestatic liver diseases. *J Hepatol*. 2009; 51(2): 237–67.

13. Mettang T. Pruritus in renal disease. Chapter 5 in: Carstens E, Akiyama T, eds. *Itch: Mechanisms and Treatment*. Boca Raton, FL: CRC Press; 2014. Available at //www.ncbi.nlm.nih.gov/books/NBK200924/. Accessed October 23, 2016.

14. Narita I, Alchi B, Omori K, et al. Etiology and prognostic significance of severe uremic pruritus in chronic hemodialysis patients. *Kidney Int*. 2006; 69(9): 1626–32.

15. Cheng SP, Lee JJ, Liu TP, et al. Parathyroidectomy improves symptomatology and quality of life in patients with secondary hyperparathyroidism. *Surgery*. 2014; 155(2): 320–8.

16. Tăranu T, Toader S, Eşanu I, Toader MP. Pruritus in the elderly: pathophysiological, clinical, laboratory and therapeutic approach. *Rev Med Chir Soc Med Nat*. 2014; 118(1): 33–8.

17. Sampogna F, Frontani M, Baliva G, et al. Quality of life and psychological distress in patients with cutaneous lymphoma. *Br J Dermatol*. 2009; 160(4): 815–22.

18. Jiménez Gallo D, Albarrán Planelles C, Linares Barrios M, Fernández Anguita MJ, Márquez Enríquez J, Rodríguez Mateos ME. Treatment of pruritus in early-stage hypopigmented mycosis fungoides with aprepitant. *Dermatol Ther*. 2014; 27(3): 178–82.

19. Kaushik S, Cerci FB, Miracle J, et al. Chronic pruritus in HIV-positive patients in the southeastern United States: its prevalence and effect on quality of life. *J Am Acad Dermatol*. 2014; 70(4): 659–64.

20. Serling SLC, Leslie K, Maurer T. Approach to pruritus in the adult HIV-positive patient. *Semin Cutan Med Surg*. 2011; 30: 101–6.

21. Dhand A, Aminoff MJ. The neurology of itch. *Brain*. 2014; 137(2): 313–22.

22. Tey HL, Wallengren J, Yosipovitch G. Psychosomatic factors in pruritus. *Clin Dermatol*. 2013; 31: 31–40.

23. Patel T, Yosipovitch G. Therapy of pruritus. *Expert Opin Pharmacother*. 2010; 11(10): 1673–82.

24. Larkin P. Pruritus, fever, and sweats. In: Ferrell BR, Coyle N, Paice J, eds. *Oxford Textbook of Palliative Nursing*. 4th ed. Oxford: Oxford University Press; 2015:325–40.

25. Rika S, Takahiro S, Ayumi T, Kazumi S, Hiroo Y. Anti-pruritic effects of topical crotamiton, capsaicin, and a corticosteroid on pruritogen-induced scratching behavior. *Exp Dermatol*. 2012; 21(3): 201–4.

26. Phan NQ, Lotts T, Antal A, Bernhard JD, Ständer S. Systemic kappa opioid receptor agonists in the treatment of chronic pruritus: a literature review. *Acta Derm Venereol*, 2012; 92: 555–60.

26. Feramisco JD, Berger TG, Steinhoff M. Innovative management of pruritus. *Dermatol Clin*. 2010; 28: 467–78.

27. Kremer AE, Bolier R, van Dijk R, Oude Elferink RP, Beuers U. Advances in pathogenesis and management of pruritus in cholestasis. *Dig Dis*. 2014; 32(5): 637–45.

28. Yue J, Jiao S, Xiao Y, Ren W, Zhao T, Meng J. Comparison of pregabalin with ondansetron in treatment of uraemic pruritus in dialysis patients: a prospective, randomized, double-blind study. *Int Urol Nephrol*. Epub 2014 Aug 7. doi: 10.1007/s11255-014-0795-x

29. To THM, Clark K, Lam L, Shelby-James T, Currow DC. The role of ondansetron in the management of cholestatic or uremic pruritus: systematic review. *J Pain Symptom Manage*. 2012; 44(5): 725–30.

30. Viegas LP, Ferreira MB, Kaplan AP. The maddening itch: an approach to chronic urticaria. *J Investig Allergol Clin Immunol*. 2014; 24(1): 1–5.

31. Parés A, Herrera M, Avilés J, Sanz M, Mas A. Treatment of resistant pruritus from cholestasis with albumin dialysis: combined analysis of patients from three centers. *J Hepatol*. 2010; 53(2): 307–12.

32. Chang FY, Lu CL. Hiccup: mystery, nature and treatment. *J Neurogastroenterol Motil*. 2012; 18(2): 123–30.

33. Regnard C. Dysphagia, dyspepsia, and hiccup. In: Hanks G, Cherny NI, Christakis NA, Fallon M, Kaasa S, Portenoy RK, eds. *Oxford Textbook of Palliative Medicine*. 4th ed. New York, NY: Oxford University Press; 2011:812–32.

34. Moretto EN, Wee B, Wiffen PJ, Murchison AG. Interventions for treating persistent and intractable hiccups in adults. *Cochrane Database Syst Rev*. 2013; 31: 1.

35. Phillips RA. The management of hiccups in terminally ill patients. *Nurs Times*. 2005; 101(31): 32–3.

36. Bredenoord AJ. Management of belching, hiccups, and aerophagia. *Clin Gastroenterol Hepatol*. 2013; 11(1): 6–12.

37. Kang JH, Hui D, Kim MJ, et al. Corticosteroid rotation to alleviate dexamethasone-induced hiccup: a case series at a single institution. *J Pain Symptom Manage*. 2014; 43(3): 625–30.

38. Marinella MA. Diagnosis and management of hiccups in the patient with advanced cancer. *J Support Oncol*. 2009; 7(4): 122.

39. Peacock ME. Transient hiccups associated with oral dexamethasone. *Case Rep Dent*. 2013; 9;2013: 426178.

40. Petroianu GA. Treatment of hiccup by vagal maneuvers. *J Hist Neurosci*. 2014; 23: 1–14.

41. Uña E, Alonso P. High dose of prokinetics for refractory hiccups after chemotherapy or the return to a simple drug. *BMJ Case Rep*. 2013; pii: bcr2013201028. doi: 10.1136/bcr-2013-201028.

42. Wang T, Wang D. Metoclopramide for patients with intractable hiccups: a multi-center, randomized, controlled pilot study. *Intern Med J*. Epub July 29, 2014. doi: 10.1111/imj.12542.

43. Ives TJ, Fleming MF, Weart CW, Bloch D. Treatment of intractable hiccups with intramuscular haloperidol. *Am J Psychiatry*. 1985; 142(11): 1368–9.

44. Zhang C, Zhang R, Zhang S, Xu M, Zhang S. Baclofen for stroke patients with persistent hiccups: a randomized, double-blind, placebo-controlled trial. *Trials*. 2014; 15(1): 295.

45. Thompson AN, Ehret Leal J, Brzezinski WA. Olanzapine and baclofen for the treatment of intractable hiccups. *Pharmacotherapy*. 2014; 34(1): e4–8.

46. Baumann A, Weicker T, Alb I, Audibert G. Baclofen for the treatment of hiccup related to brainstem compression. *Ann Fr Anesth Reanim*. 2014; 33(1): e27–28.

47. Mirijello A, Addolorato G, D'Angelo C, et al. Baclofen in the treatment of persistent hiccup: a case series. *Int J Clin Pract*. 2013; 67(9): 918–21.

48. Thompson DF, Brooks KG. Gabapentin therapy of hiccups. *Ann Pharmacother*. 2013; 47(6): 897–903.

49. Porzio G, Aielli F, Verna L, Aloisi P, Galletti B, Ficorella C. Gabapentin in the treatment of hiccups in patients with advanced cancer: a 5-year experience. *Clin Neuropharmacol*. 2010; 33(4): 179–180.

50. Quigley C. Nifedipine for hiccups. *J Pain Symptom Manage*. 1997; 13(6): 313.

51. Stueber D, Swartz CM. Carvedilol suppresses intractable hiccups. *J Am Board Fam Med*. 2006; 19: 418–21.

52. Kaneishi K, Kawabata M. Continuous subcutaneous infusion of lidocaine for persistent hiccup in advanced cancer. *Palliat Med*. 2013; 27(3): 284–5.

53. Wilcox SK, Garry A, Johnson MJ. Novel use of amantadine: to treat hiccups. *J Pain Symptom Manage*. 2009; 38: 460–5.

54. Kang KN, Park IK, Suh JH, Leem JG, Shin JW. Ultrasound-guided pulsed radiofrequency lesioning of the phrenic nerve in a patient with intractable hiccup. *Korean J Pain*. 2010; 23: 198–201.

55. Lin YC. Acupuncture for persistent hiccups in a heart and lung transplant recipient. *J Heart Lung Transplant*. 2006; 25(1): 126.

56. Ge AX, Ryan ME, Giaccone G, Hughes MS, Pavletic SZ. Acupuncture treatment for persistent hiccups in patients with cancer. *J Altern Complement Med*. 2010; 16(7): 811.

57. Davies A, Hall S. Salivary gland dysfunction (dry mouth) in patients with advanced cancer. *Int J Palliat Nurs*. 2011; 17(10): 477–82.

58. Reisfeld G, Rosielle D, Wilson G. Fast Facts and Concepts #182. Xerostomia. Palliative Care Network of Wisconsin. Available at http://www.mypcnow. org/blank-zlal4. Accessed October 21, 2016.

59. Dahlin CM, Cohen AK. Dysphagia, xerostomia, and hiccups. In: Ferrell BR, Coyle N, Paice J, eds. *Oxford Textbook of Palliative Nursing*. 4th ed. Oxford: Oxford University Press; 2015:191–216.

60. Lalla RV, Peterson DE. Oral symptoms. In: Walsh D, Caraceni AT, Fainsinger R, et al., eds. *Palliative Medicine*. Philadelphia, PA: Saunders Elsevier; 2009:937–46.

61. Wolff A, Fox PD, Porter S, Konttinen Y. Established and novel approaches for the management of hyposalivation and xerostomia. *Curr Pharm Design*. 2012; 18: 5515–21.

62. Bobb B, Lyckholm L, Coyne P. Fever and sweats. In: Walsh D, Caraceni AT, Fainsinger R, et al., eds. *Palliative Medicine*. Philadelphia, PA: Saunders Elsevier; 2009:890–3.

63. Strickland M, Stovsky E. Fast Facts and Concepts #256. Fever at the end of life. 2012. Palliative Care Network of Wisconsin. Available at http://www. mypcnow.org/blank-lu7n4. Accessed October 21, 2016.

64. Bourdeanu L, Hein MJ, Liu E. Insomnia. In: Ferrell BR, Coyle N, Paice J, eds. *Oxford Textbook of Palliative Nursing*. 4th ed. Oxford: Oxford University Press; 2015:404–10.

65. Arnold R, Miller M, Mehta R. Fast Facts and Concepts #101. Insomnia: patient assessment. 202015. 2nd ed. Palliative Care Network of Wisconsin. Available at http://www.mypcnow.org/blank-xwnba. Accessed October 21, 2016.

66. Khoshknabi DS. Sleep problems and nightmares. In: Walsh D, Caraceni AT, Fainsinger R, et al., eds. *Palliative Medicine*. Philadelphia, PA: Saunders Elsevier; 2009:965–72.

67. Walia HK, Shalhoub G, Ramsammy V, Thornton JD, Auckley D. Symptoms of restless leg syndrome in a palliative care population: frequency and impact. *J Palliat Care*. 2013; 29: 201–16.

68. Davis M, Goforth H. Fighting insomnia and battling lethargy: the yin and yang of palliative care. *Curr Oncol Rep*. 2014; 16(4): 377–95.

69. Arnold R, Miller M, Mehta R. Fast Facts and Concepts #105. Insomnia: drug therapies. Palliative Care Network of Wisconsin. Available at http://www. mypcnow.org/blank-vsd01. Accessed October 21, 2016.

Chapter 5

Nausea and Vomiting

Maureen Lynch

Key Points

- When medications are used as part of the management plan, the advanced practice registered nurse (APRN) must consider the pharmacologic class of the drug and use only one per class.
- The use of appropriate nonpharmacologic interventions specific to the patient's condition is part of the APRN's approach to the management of nausea and vomiting.

Physiology

The vomiting center responds to input from afferent pathways that include the chemoreceptor trigger zone (CTZ), the vagus nerve, the cerebral cortex, and the vestibular system. The cerebral cortex signals the vomiting center via the midbrain. Stimuli include anticipation, fear, and memories (e.g., anticipatory vomiting) as well as signals from the senses, such as disturbing sights, smells, or pain. The vomiting center also responds to vestibular input via the inner ear, mediated by histamine and acetylcholine. Motion, certain medications, and changes in intracranial pressure may trigger this pathway. With threshold stimulation of these afferent pathways, the vomiting center triggers the efferent pathways that coordinate the complex sequence of powerful and sustained contractions of the abdominal muscles and diaphragm and relaxation of pyloric and duodenal sphincters that forces expulsion of gastric contents via the mouth.[1–6]

Less information exists about the physiological pathways that control nausea. While vomiting is a reflex controlled by lower brain structures, nausea seems to require consciousness and cerebral function.[3] The changes in gastric motility are accompanied by a decrease in gastric acid levels and release of cortisol, beta endorphins, epinephrine, and norepinephrine, causing nausea, pallor, cold sweats, tachypnea, tachycardia, and increased salivation.[1,2,5] The CTZ plays a role in the development of nausea through its effect on gastrointestinal motility, taste aversion, and food intake.[1]

Etiology

Nausea, vomiting, and retching are distinct phenomena that may be experienced acutely, chronically, independently, simultaneously, or sequentially. In palliative care, the etiologies of nausea and vomiting (N/V) are often multifactorial and may be related to underlying disease and/or comorbidities, treatment effects, or debility.[3] A primary etiology of N/V can be identified in most patients.[3]

N/V are often experienced in relation to other symptoms. Studies of N/V in oncology describe clustering of nausea, vomiting, loss of appetite, taste changes, weight loss, and fatigue.[7,8] Table 5.1 outlines common etiologies of N/V to be considered in formulating a differential diagnosis.

Assessment

Identifying the presence of the symptom(s) is the first step in assessment. The subjectivity of nausea makes it harder to identify than vomiting. The patient's report of N/V, either spontaneously or in the clinical interview, is a frequent method of symptom identification. Routine screening for common symptoms using symptom inventory tools such as the Memorial Symptom Assessment Scale or the Edmonton Symptom Assessment System is another method of symptom identification.[11]

The effects of the N/V on function and quality of life are essential parts of the assessment. N/V symptoms often change eating patterns and are accompanied by diminished physical functioning and self-care capacity. In turn, social isolation, uncertainty, and worry about how N/V affect day-to-day life, medical therapies, family caregivers, and survival add to symptom distress.

Patient diaries and journals may aid in understanding the patient's perception of and response to N/V. There are also specific assessment tools for evaluating N/V. The Morrow Assessment of Nausea and Vomiting (MANE) and the Rhodes Index of Nausea and Vomiting (INVR) enhance the patient's report of the symptom characteristics. Other tools, such as Functional Living Index-Emesis and Osoba Nausea and Emesis Module, describe the effect of the symptoms on function and well-being[10,12–14] (Table 5.2).

Management Strategies

The goal of antiemetic therapy is to modify or alleviate the patient's experience of N/V by reducing the incidence and severity of both, addressing symptom-related distress, and modifying or eliminating the cause if possible. Broad categories of interventions include patient and family education, psychosocial and spiritual support, behavioral and lifestyle changes, medications, invasive procedures, and etiology-directed therapies. Table 5.3 summarizes management approaches.

Table 5.1 Common Etiologies of Nausea and Vomiting

Gastrointestinal	Drug-induced
• Ascites	• Antibiotics
• Adhesions	• Anticonvulsants
• Biliary obstruction	• Aspirin and NSAIDs
• Cholecystitis	• Chemotherapy
• Constipation	• Digoxin
• Gastric irritation/distention	• Iron supplements
• Gastroparesis	• Opioids
• Gastric outlet obstruction	• Theophylline
• Gastric reflux	**Radiation-induced**
• Hepatitis	• Esophagus
• Hepatic capsular distention	• Abdominal
• Intestinal obstruction	• Pelvic
• Irritable bowel	• Brain
• Intra-abdominal cancers:	
Colon, pancreas, ovarian, gastric, esophageal	
• Peritoneal carcinomatosis	
• Pancreatitis	
• Gastric or duodenal ulcers	
Metabolic	**Increased intracranial pressure**
• Fluid and electrolyte imbalances:	• Cerebral edema
Hypercalcemia	• Intracranial tumor
Hyper/hyponatremia	• Intracranial bleeding
• Dehydration	• Skull metastases
• Adrenocortical insufficiency	• Carcinomatous meningitis
• Liver failure	
• Renal failure	
• Diabetic ketoacidosis	
• Pregnancy	
Infections	**Psychological**
• *Candida* esophagitis	• Fear
• Gastroenteritis	• Anxiety
• Sepsis	
Vestibular	**Pharyngea**
• Motion sickness	• Chronic cough
• Ménière syndrome	• Oropharyngeal secretions
• Vestibular problems	

Adapted from reference 9. Sources: references 1–3, 5, 10.

61

Pharmacologic Interventions

There are seven classes of drugs used in antiemetic therapy: dopamine receptor antagonists, including prokinetics and neuroleptics (antipsychotics), serotonin receptor antagonists, antihistamines, anticholinergics, corticosteroids, cannabinoids, and NK$_1$ receptor antagonists (Table 5.4). Understanding the action and side effects of the different antiemetics aids

Table 5.2 Assessment of Nausea and Vomiting

	Nausea	Vomiting
General	*Knowing the Patient* Demographics: age, gender, race, employment, education, place of residence, socioeconomics, health insurance Spiritual: values/beliefs, faith community, practices, rituals, restrictions Psychosocial: marital status, sexual preference, culture, coping, social supports, substance use concerns, past experience with health-related issues Current quality-of-life concerns	
Health status	Current diagnosis; prognosis; disease course and trajectory, including past and current therapies; patient's understanding of disease status; goals of care Past medical history, including history of nausea or vomiting and effective therapies	
Symptom experience	Patient description: nausea, upset stomach, queasiness, sick stomach, other	Description of "throwing up," "upchucking," "barfing": volume, color, content of emesis
Severity	0 none–10 worst; mild/moderate/severe intensity; episodes per day/week/month; intermittent or constant	Frequency per day/week; intensity of vomiting
Duration and pattern	Onset; pattern and timing of occurrence	
Modulating factors	What makes your nausea or vomiting better or worse? (e.g., time of day, medications, eating, activity, bowel function)	
Distress/Impact	*Meaning of symptom; interference with function and quality of life:* What and how much are you able to eat or drink? What concerns you most about the nausea and/or vomiting? What worries do you have about what is causing it? Do you have an inability to eat or drink? Are you able to eat with family/friends? What effects does it have on energy and activity? Are there family concerns? What have been the effects on treatments? Have you had concerns about your appetite/weight in the past? - Overweight? - Underweight? - History of anorexia/bulimia?	

Associated symptoms	Fever, cough, oropharyngeal secretions, dizziness, headaches, vision changes, anorexia, dysgeusia, dysphagia, abdominal pain, bloating, abdominal distention, heartburn, hiccups, constipation, diarrhea, weight changes
Physical examination	Temperature
	Weight: if available, comparison to past weights is helpful
	Neurological: level of consciousness; cognition, balance, cranial nerve deficits
	Oropharynx: mucositis, secretions, infection, obstruction
	Blood pressure and pulse: sitting, lying, standing to assess for postural hypotension from fluid imbalance
	Abdomen: distention, bowel sounds, tenderness, masses
	Rectal exam: fecal impaction
Diagnostic tests: As indicated by history and physical findings and patient's health status and goals of care	Laboratory tests for renal and hepatic function, electrolytes, calcium
	Complete blood count
	Blood or urine cultures if infection is suspected
	Therapeutic drug level monitoring, if appropriate (digoxin, theophylline, etc.)
	Radiological studies
	Brain scans if CNS pathology suspected
	Chest x-ray if pneumonia suspected
	Plain film of abdomen to assess for obstruction or constipation
	CT scan of abdomen to assess for obstruction, other pathologies
	Endoscopic evaluation to assess for reflux, esophagitis, obstruction

From references 1, 2, 9, 10, 12.

Table 5.3 Approaches to Managing Nausea and Vomiting in Palliative Care

Identification and management of etiology and contributing symptoms	
Patient and family education	Likely causes of nausea and vomiting for this patient
	Goals for symptom management
	Directions re: specific interventions and self-monitoring, including emergent situations
	Information about how to contact care team
Psychosocial and spiritual support	Acknowledge the psychological, social, cultural, and religious impact of nausea and vomiting as appropriate for patient and family
	Refer to social worker, chaplain, or psychiatric support, if needed
Nutrition counseling	Mouth care[a]
	Small, frequent meals or snacks[a]
	Maintain fluid intake but limit fluids with meals[a]
	Pleasant eating environment[a]
	Eat bland, cool temperature foods[a]
	Avoid salty, sweet, spicy foods[a]
	Use enriched and fortified foods to increased calories and protein.
	Use of commercial oral liquid nutritional supplements
	Consultation with qualified nutritionist
Cognitive-behavioral therapies	Includes relaxation, imagery, distraction, self-hypnosis[b]
Integrative therapies	Acupuncture[b]
	Acupressure[c]
	Ginger[c]
	Aromatherapy[c]
Medications	See Table 5.4.
Artificial hydration and nutrition	Generally not tolerated or beneficial in patients who have end-stage disease. Individualized goals of the therapy need to be considered.
	May benefit patients with early-stage disease who have temporary limitations in oral intake or those with GI malfunctions but high performance status
Invasive procedures	For obstructions: surgery, venting gastrostomy tubes, stents

[a]Expert opinion; [b]Limited data to support use; [c]Mixed or no data to support use.
From references 1, 2, 10, 15–21.

in medication selection.[3,22,23] Regardless of the approach, if initial therapies are unsuccessful, adding or changing to an agent from a different class of antiemetics may be beneficial. The simultaneous use of more than one agent from each class is generally avoided to prevent overlapping side effects or toxicities.[3] The concurrent use of agents from different classes may be beneficial.

Table 5.4 Commonly Used Antiemetics

Drug	Suggested Doses	Primary Neuroreceptor Affinity	Common Use	Side Effects/Comments
DOPAMINE RECEPTOR ANTAGONISTS				
Prokinetic agent Metoclopramide	Oral, ODT, IV: 10–20 mg, q 6–12h	Moderate D_2 (primarily in GI tract) Low $5HT_3$ (only at high doses)	Gastroparesis Ileus in absence of complete obstruction	EPS; esophageal spasm; colic in GI tract obstruction; prolonged half-life in renal failure QT prolongation Do not use in complete bowel obstruction
Butyrophenone Haloperidol	Oral: 0.5–5 mg q 8–12h IV: 0.5–1 mg q 6–8h	High D_2	Chemical and/or metabolic nausea Bowel obstruction	Less sedating than phenothiazines May cause QT prolongation, EPS, neuroleptic malignant syndrome Dose reduction may be needed in hepatic insufficiency
Phenothiazine Prochlorperazine	Oral: 5–10 mg q 6–8h PR: 25 mg q 12h IV: 10 mg q 6h Max dose: 40 mg/24 h	Moderate D_2 Low H_1	Chemical and/or metabolic nausea	EPS, headache, dry mouth, hypotension, drowsiness, QT prolongation
Chlorpromazine	Oral: 10–25 q 6h IV: 12.5–25 mg q 6–12h	Moderate D_2 Low H_1	Chemical and/or metabolic nausea	More sedating than prochlorperazine EPS, QT prolongation
Atypical Antipsychotic Olanzapine	Oral: 2.5–10 mg q 12–24h	D_{1-4}, $5HT_3$, H_1	Refractory nausea/ vomiting	Sedation; hyperglycemia; reduced seizure threshold Associated with weight gain and improved appetite Lower risk of EPS QT prolongation

(continued)

Table 5.4 Continued

Drug	Suggested Doses	Primary Neuroreceptor Affinity	Common Use	Side Effects/Comments
CORTICOSTEROID				
Dexamethasone	Oral: 2–4 mg q 6–24h IV: 2–4 mg q 6–24h	Possibly reduces release of serotonin or activation of corticosteroid receptors in the CNS	Cerebral edema Intracranial tumors Chemotherapy-induced nausea Bowel obstruction	Insomnia, anxiety, euphoria; perirectal burning with IV administration; GI upset Metabolic effects: glycemic control, infection risk
SEROTONIN ANTAGONISTS				
Ondansetron	Oral/ODT/IV: 4–8 mg q 8–12h	High $5HT_3$ Both peripherally and centrally	Chemotherapy-induced nausea	Constipation Headache
Granisetron	Oral/IV: 1 mg q 12h or 2 mg q 24h Transdermal patch: 3.1 mg/24 h (lasts 7 days)		Abdominal radiation therapy Postop GI irritants	Diarrhea Mild sedation QT prolongation
CANNABINOIDS				
Dronabinol	2–10 mg q 8–12h Contains sesame oil	CB_1	Second-line antiemetic	Sedation, dizziness, disorientation, concentration difficulties, dysphoria, hypotension, dry mouth, tachycardia
Nabilone	1–2 mg q 8–12h (max dose 6 mg/day)	CB_1	Second-line antiemetic	
ANTICHOLINERGICS				
Hyoscyamine	Oral/IV: 0.125–0.25 mg q 4h as needed up to 1.5 mg/day	mAChR (in the vomiting center and peripherally)	Intestinal obstruction Peritoneal irritation Increased intracranial Pressure Excess secretions Motion sickness	Dry mouth, ileus, urinary retention, blurred vision, agitation
Scopolamine	Transdermal: 1.5 mg q 72h (lasts 72 h)			Onset of effect is up to 24 h.

ANTIHISTAMINES

Drug	Dose	Receptor	Indication	Side effects
Promethazine	Oral, PR, or IV: 12.5–25 mg q6–8h (max dose 100 mg/day)	High H_1 Low D_2 Low mAChR	Motion sickness Increased intracranial pressure	Sedation Dry mouth Constipation Dizziness Confusion Blurred vision
Cyclizine	Oral: 25–50 mg q6–8h (max dose 200 mg/day)	H_1		
Diphenhydramine	Oral/IV: 12.5–50 mg q6–8h			

BENZODIAZEPINE

Drug	Dose	Receptor	Indication	Side effects
Lorazepam	Oral/IV: 0.5–1 mg q6–24h	GABA	Anxiety Not FDA approved as antiemetic	Sedation, amnesia, delirium, Depression. Reduce dose in renal or hepatic insufficiency

OTHER

Drug	Dose	Receptor	Indication	Side effects
Octreotide (somatostatin analogue)	SC: 100–150 mg q8h IV continuous infusion: 0.2–0.9 mg/day IM depot: 20–30 mg q3–4 weeks	Somatostatin receptors in brain, pituitary, GI tract	Bowel obstruction. Reduces peristalsis and intestinal secretions	Pain at injection site; worsening GI symptoms. Reduce dose in renal or hepatic insufficiency.
Mirtazapine (antidepressant)	Oral: 7.5–30 mg at bedtime	$5HT_3$, H_1, mAChR	Gastroparesis	Increased appetite; weight gain, somnolence

ODT, oral disintegrating tablet; D_2, dopamine; H_1, histamine; $5HT_3$, serotonin; CB_1, cannabinoid; mAChR, muscarinic acetylcholine receptors; EPS, extrapyramidal side effects. Adapted from reference 9. Sources: references 1–3, 10, 22–29.

Dopamine receptor antagonist (D_2) antiemetics are active at the CTZ and in the gut.[24] Commonly used drugs in this class are metoclopramide and neuroleptics, such as prochlorperazine, chlorpromazine, haloperidol, and olanzapine. Gastroparesis is a common cause of N/V in palliative care. Thus, the pro-motility effect of metoclopramide on the upper gastrointestinal tract and its activity at the CTZ make it a useful first-line antiemetic.[3,22,23] However, it should be avoided in patients with complete bowel obstruction.[3,22]

Extrapyramidal side effects that range from mild to moderate akathisia (subjective sense of restlessness to motor restlessness), parkinsonian-like changes (masked faces, resting tremor, cogwheel rigidity, shuffling gait, bradykinesia), dystonias (involuntary contraction of major muscles [e.g., torticollis, oculogyric crisis]), and tardive dyskinesia (characterized by lip smacking, rhythmic tongue and/or body movements, grimacing) may be associated with dopamine receptor antagonist use. Management of extra-pyramidal symptoms includes discontinuing the drug or reducing the dose. Co-administering a benzodiazepine, a beta-blocker, or an anticholinergic may temporarily reduce akathisia and dystonia.[30]

Selective $5HT_3$ (serotonin receptor subtype) receptor antagonists (e.g., ondansetron and granisetron) work on receptors in the gut, the CTZ, and the vomiting center. They are primarily used for management of N/V caused by chemotherapy and radiation therapy that affects digestive system organs, and in the postoperative setting. Constipation and QT prolongation are potential side effects.[1,3,26] Cost may be a factor in access to these medications.[1]

Antihistamines block H_1 receptor activity at the CTZ and the vomiting center. They are primarily used to manage N/V caused by vestibular stimulation (e.g., motion sickness, raised intracranial pressure). Promethazine, cyclizine, meclizine, and diphenhydramine are commonly used agents. Sedation and anticholinergic side effects may limit use. The elderly and frail may be more prone to delirium as a side effect.[1,3]

Anticholinergic agents are primarily used as antiemetics in combination with other antiemetics for control of N/V associated with dizziness and movement and bowel obstruction[10,23] resulting in decreased peristaltic tone and movement and reduced intestinal secretions.[10,26] Hyoscyamine and scopolamine are commonly used drugs in this class.

Corticosteroids are often used in antiemetic regimens for chemotherapy-induced N/V, for symptom management in bowel obstruction, and in treatment of raised intracranial pressure. Concerns about gastric irritation, glycemic control, infection risk, proximal muscle weakness with long-term use, and dysphoria and/or delirium may limit their use.[3,26]

Cannabinoids' activity at the CB_1 receptors in the central and peripheral nervous systems is thought to be the basis of their antiemetic effect. Dronabinol and nabilone are approved by the US Food and Drug Administration (FDA) for use in chemotherapy-induced N/V.[26,31] Neurokinin-1 receptor antagonists are FDA-approved for use in acute chemotherapy-associated N/V and in the postoperative setting. Drugs in this class are aprepitant and fosaprepitant. Benzodiazepines act on gamma-aminobutyric acid (GABA) in the cerebral cortex. They are effective in managing anxiety associated with N/V but do not have antiemetic activity.[3,26] Side effects of sedation and amnesia may limit use.

Mirtazapine, a tetracyclic antidepressant, has activity as a $5HT_3$, H_1, and muscarinic receptor antagonist. Reports of its antiemetic effect in diabetic gastroparesis and idiopathic nausea are indicative of a prokinetic effect that needs further study in the palliative care population.[3,26]

Management of Opioid-Induced N/V

Opioid-induced N/V may result from gastroparesis, constipation, CTZ stimulation, and/or vestibular stimulation. Managing associated symptoms, such as constipation, and consideration of changing the opioid or its route of administration when possible are reasonable management strategies. Although there are no specific antiemetic recommendations in the literature, empiric use of antiemetics, especially with initial use of the opioid, also seems reasonable.[14]

Conclusion

Successful management of these complex symptoms requires an ongoing comprehensive assessment to describe the patient's experience and associated factors, formulate a symptom diagnosis based on an understanding of likely etiologies, and use appropriate nonpharmacologic and pharmacologic management strategies based on best evidence, expert opinion, and patient acceptability.

References

1. Tipton J. Nausea and vomiting. In: Yarbro CH, Wujcik D, Gobel BH, eds. *Cancer Symptom Management*. Burlington, MA: Jones and Bartlett, Inc.; 2014:213–33.

2. Del Fabbro E. Palliative care: assessment and management of nausea and vomiting. Up-to-Date®. 2016. Available at https://www.uptodate.com/contents/palliative-care-assessment-and-management-of-nausea-and-vomiting?source=search_result&search=nausea%20and%20vomiting%20palliative&selectedTitle=1~150. Accessed October 23, 2016.

3. Glare P, Miller J, Nikolova T, Tickoo R. Treating nausea and vomiting in palliative care: a review. *Clin Interventions Aging*. 2011; 6: 243–59.

4. Parker LA, Rock EM, Limebeer CL. Regulation of nausea and vomiting by cannabinoids. *Br J Pharmacol*. 2011; 163: 1411–22.

5. Longstreth GF. Approach to adult nausea and vomiting. Up-to-Date®. 2016. Available at https://www.uptodate.com/contents/approach-to-the-adult-with-nausea-and-vomiting?source=search_result&search=nausea%20and%20vomiting%20adult&selectedTitle=1~150. Accessed October 23, 2016.

6. Howard HS, Smith JM, Smith AR. Pathophysiology of nausea/vomiting in palliative medicine. *Ann Palliat Med*. 2012. Available at http://apm.amegroups.com/article/view/995/1260. Accessed October 23, 2016.

7. Molassiotis A, Farrell C, Bourne K, et al. An exploratory study to clarify the cluster of symptoms predictive of chemotherapy related nausea using random forest remodeling. *J Pain Symptom Manage*. 2012; 44(5): 692–703.

8. Cherwin, CH. Gastrointestinal symptom representation in cancer symptoms cluster: a review of the literature. *Oncol Nurs Forum*. 2012; 39(2): 157–65.

9. Hawkins R, Lynch M. Nausea and vomiting. In: Dahlin CM, Lynch M, eds. *Core Curriculum for the Advanced Practice Hospice and Palliative Registered Nurse*. 2nd ed. Pittsburgh, PA: Hospice and Palliative Nursing Association; 2013.

10. Chow K, Cogan, D, Mun S. Nausea and vomiting. In: Ferrell BR, Coyle N, Paice J., eds. *Oxford Textbook of Palliative Nursing*. 4th ed. New York, NY: Oxford University Press Inc., 2015: 175–90.

11. Bookbinder M, McHugh ME. Symptom management in palliative care and end of life. *Nurs Clin North Am*. 2010; 45(3): 271–327.

12. Rhodes VA, McDaniel RW. Nausea, vomiting, retching: complex problems in palliative care. *CA Cancer J Clinicians*. 2001; 51(4): 232–48.

13. Wood JM, Chapman K, Eilers J. Tools for assessing nausea, vomiting, retching. *Cancer Nurs*. 2011; 34(1): E14–24.

14. Saxby C, Acroyd R, Callin S, Mayland C. How should we measure emesis in palliative care? *Palliat Med*. 2007; 21: 369–83.

15. Oncology Nursing Society. Putting Evidence into Practice. Chemotherapy-induced nausea and vomiting. 2016. Available at https://www.ons.org/practice-resources/pep/chemotherapy-induced-nausea-and-vomiting/chemotherapy-induced-nausea-and. Accessed October 23, 2016.

16. Holmer Patterson P, Wengstrom Y. Acupuncture prior to surgery to minimize postoperative nausea and vomiting: a systematic review. *J Clin Nurs*. 2012; 21(13–14): 1799–805.

17. Lee EJ, Frazier SK. The efficacy of acupressure for symptom management: a systematic review. *J Pain Symptom Manage*. 2011; 42(4): 589–603.

18. Molassiotis A, Russell WH, Breckons M, et al. The effectiveness, and cost effectiveness of acupressure for the control and management of chemotherapy related acute and delayed nausea: assessment of nausea in chemotherapy research (ANCHoR), a randomized controlled trial. *Health Technol Assess*. 2013; 17(26): 1–114.

19. Lee J, Oh, H. Ginger as an antiemetic modality for chemotherapy-induced nausea and vomiting: a systematic review and meta-analysis. *Oncol Nurs Forum*. 2013: 40(2): 163–70.

20. Dev R, Dalal S, Bruera E. Is there a role for parenteral nutrition or hydration at end of life? *Curr Op Support Palliat Care*. 2012; 6(3): 365–70.

21. Hospice and Palliative Nursing Association. *HPNA Position Statement: Artificial Hydration and Nutrition in Advanced Illness*. 2011. Available at http://hpna.advancingexpertcare.org/wp-content/uploads/2015/08/Artificial-Nutrition-and-Hydration-in-Advanced-Illness.pdf. Accessed October 23, 2016.

22. Benze G, Alt-Epping B, Geyer A, Nauck F. Treatment of nausea and vomiting with prokinetics and neuroleptics in palliative care patients (English version). *Der Schmerz*. 2012; 26: 500–14.

23. Davis MP, Hallerberg G. A systematic review of the treatment of nausea and/or vomiting in cancer unrelated to chemotherapy or radiation. *J Pain Symptom Manage*. 2010; 39(4): 756–67.

24. Jordan K, Schmoll HJ, Aapro MS. Comparative activity of antiemetic drugs. *Crit Rev Hematol Oncol*. 2007; 61: 162–75.

25. Pommer E. Olanzapine: palliative medicine update. *Am J Hospice Palliat Med*. 2012; 30(1): 75–82.

26. Benze G, Geyer A, Alt-Epping B, Nauck F. Treatment of nausea and vomiting with 5HT3 receptor antagonists, steroids, antihistamines, anticholinergics, somatastatin analogs, benzodiazepines and cannabinoids in palliative care patients [English version]. *Der Schmerz.* 2012: 26: 481–99.

27. Ripamonti C, Mercandante S. Pathophysiology and management of malignant bowel obstructions. In: Hanks G, Cherny NI, Christakis NA, Kassa S, Portemoy R, eds. *Textbook of Palliative Medicine.* 4th ed. New York, NY: Oxford University Press; 2010:850–63.

28. Mercandante S, Porzio G. Octreotide for malignant bowel obstruction: twenty years after. *Crit Rev Oncol Hematol.* 2012; 83(3): 388–92.

29. Pommer E. Role of haloperidol in palliative medicine: an update. *Am J Hospice Palliat Med.* 2012; 29(4): 295–301.

30. Marder S, Stroup TS. Pharmacotherapy for schizophrenia: side effect management. Up-to-Date®. 2016. Available at https://www.uptodate.com/contents/pharmacotherapy-for-schizophrenia-side-effect-management?source=search_result&search=schizophrenia%20treatment&selectedTitle=4~150. Accessed October 23, 2016.

31. Howard P, Twycross R, Schuster J, et al. Cannabinoids. *J Pain Symptom Manage.* 2013; 46(1): 142–9.

Chapter 6

Anxiety

Maria Gatto, Patricia Thomas, and Ann Berger

Key Points

- Anxiety is a universal, subjective, and objective life experience that crosses all eight palliative care domains of the National Consensus Project for Quality Palliative Care (NCP) *Clinical Practice Guidelines*.
- Anxiety and chronic diseases are interchangeable in their causal relationship: chronic diseases can exacerbate symptoms of anxiety, and anxiety disorders can lead to chronic diseases.

Introduction

Anxiety is a multidimensional, subjective, and objective experience with manifestations of physical, affective, behavioral, and cognitive responses.[1] These include feelings of worry, apprehension, tension, and nervousness that are unpleasant and distressful, but they are a common response for patients and family members when faced with a serious diagnosis.

Anxiety is a natural and expected part of the coping process that helps us adapt to everyday concerns. However, extreme distressful anxiety can impair daily function, causing disability and disruptions in quality of life for patients, family, and caregivers.[2] Specific differentiation between anxiety as a normal response and a specific diagnostic criterion that requires professional intervention and treatment is outlined according to the fifth edition of *The Diagnostic and Statistical Manual of Mental Disorders* (DSM-V-TR).[3] The experience of apparent uncontrollable physical, affective, behavioral, and cognitive symptoms having no specific stimulus warrants consideration of a pathological disorder. Anxiety disorders are categorized according to criteria and range in complexity and severity from panic attacks, acute stress disorder, generalized anxiety disorder, social anxiety disorders, phobias, obsessive–compulsive disorder, post-traumatic stress disorder, anxiety secondary to a medical condition, and substance-induced anxiety disorders.[3]

Common situations, medical conditions, medications, and substances are associated with and can cause nonspecific anxiety symptoms.[4] Existential and psychosocial concerns increase anxiety when a person is faced with mortality; long-term or permanent disability; loss of control; family and financial crisis; loss of meaning, hope, and purpose; and religious or spiritual crisis. There

Table 6.1 Associated Causes and Mimics of Anxiety	
Acute emotional disruption	Interpersonal stresses
Anger	Legitimate worries and concerns
Anxiety disorders	Loss of control
Coping style (ineffective patterns or behaviors)	Pain
Delirium	Physical symptoms
Fear	Medication side effects
Financial concerns	Spiritual and existential crisis
Grief and bereavement	Withdrawal states
From references 1, 4, 5.	

is also considerable overlap and confusion among the anxiety, depression, and delirium that commonly arise as part of an illness trajectory and that can either lead, progress to, or continue in a vicious downward cycle when not recognized and treated appropriately (Table 6.1).

Definitions and the Distress Continuum

Any serious illness is a life-altering experience. This is an extremely fragile period filled with fear and anxiety. Information, communication, and overall psychosocial support are priority needs for the patient's mental well-being.

Anxiety ranges from normal adjustment issues to syndromes that meet the diagnostic criteria for mental disorders. It occurs on a continuum of increasing levels and severity of psychosocial distress, ranging from normal adjustment to adjustment disorders and subthreshold mental disorders to diagnosable mental disorders (Tables 6.2, 6.3, and 6.4).[6–8]

Life-Transforming Change

Life-transforming change can result from the illness experience. Some patients experience a total paradigm shift, where unanticipated discovery of personal abilities and untapped resources helps the patient overcome the challenges of serious and advanced illness and life challenges outside of serious and advanced illness. With this shift, the patient's life is taken to a previously unknown level where he or she experiences a more fulfilling, purposeful, and meaningful life, with greater depth psychosocially and spiritually (Table 6.5).

Screening and Assessment

A variety of screening tools are available based on the patient's presentation. Screening may include a brief, self-report questionnaire method. The patient's score establishes the level and severity of distress to guide the next steps. If the distress is high, a referral for an in-depth psychosocial assessment by an appropriate mental health professional is made.[10]

Table 6.2 Summary of Psychosocial Distress Definitions

Normal adjustment	Ongoing life processes and coping responses associated with living with a serious illness: • Manage emotional distress • Solve specific cancer-related problems • Gain mastery or control over cancer-related life events
Psychosocial distress	Extends along a continuum ranging from: • Common normal feelings (vulnerability, sadness, and fear) to problems that are disabling (i.e., depression, anxiety, panic) • Feeling isolated • Spiritual crisis Unpleasant experience of: • Emotional, psychological, social, or spiritual nature that interferes with the ability to cope with treatment for the illness
Adjustment disorders	A diagnostic category of the fifth revised edition of the American Psychiatric Association's *Diagnostic and Statistical Manual of Mental Disorders* (DSM-V-TR): • Reactions to an identifiable psychosocial stressor with a degree of psychopathology • Less severe than diagnosable mental disorders yet in excess of what would be expected • Result in significant impairment in social or occupational functioning (i.e., major depressive disorder, generalized anxiety disorder)
Anxiety disorders	Group of mental disorders whose common symptoms include excessive, unwarranted, often illogical anxiety, worry, fear, apprehension, and/or dread. The DSM-V-TR examples include generalized anxiety disorder, panic disorder, agoraphobia, social anxiety disorder, specific phobia, obsessive-compulsive disorder, and post-traumatic stress disorder.

From reference 8.

Communication with patients and family members, and their participation as partners in care, are key. The patient and family are part of the process since assessment is a combination of self-report and evaluation by members of the professional team. This approach to assessing caregivers' needs and strengths can improve the overall health and quality of life for both the patient and caregivers.[11] The five major components of the caregiver experience that provide insight into caregiver stress are caregiver context, primary stressors, secondary stressors, resources, and outcomes.[12]

Caregiver context addresses sociodemographic information, history of illness, and caregiving and living arrangements. Primary stressors from the patient experience are symptoms, impairments, activities of daily living, behavioral and cognitive issues, and the caregiver's subjective burden. Secondary stressors are tension and conflicts of employment, relationships, and maintaining roles and responsibility. Resources are social, financial,

Table 6.3 Anxiety and Chronic Disease Prevalence	
Medical Conditions	**Examples**
Cardiovascular	Angina, congestive heart failure, hypovolemia, mitral valve prolapse, myocardial infarction, paroxysmal atrial tachycardia
Endocrine	Carcinoid syndrome, Cushing's disease, hyperglycemia, hypoglycemia, hyperthyroidism, hypothyroidism, pheochromocytoma
Immune	HIV/AIDS
Metabolic	Anemia, hypercalcemia, hyperkalemia, hypoglycemia, hyponatremia, hyperthermia
Respiratory	Asthma, chronic obstructive pulmonary disease, hypoxia, pneumonia, pulmonary disease, pulmonary edema, pulmonary embolus
Neurological	Akathisia, encephalopathy, brain lesion, seizure disorders, post-concussion syndrome, vertigo, cerebral vascular accident, dementia
Neoplasms	Islet cell adenomas, pheochromocytoma
Cancer	Hormone-producing tumors, pheochromocytoma
From references 1, 4, 5.	

emotional, and gains from experience. Outcomes are either positive or negative health outcomes related to the caregiver.[13]

Inappropriate or incomplete awareness of cultural, religious, and spiritual beliefs or needs can lead to inappropriate and unacceptable plans of care, resulting in unnecessary and undue anxiety and distress.

To complete the comprehensive anxiety assessment processes and psychosocial spiritual screening and assessments, a physical examination is appropriate; it could reveal anxiety-associated medical conditions, emergent pathophysiology, and medications and substances whose side effects mimic anxiety.

Pharmacologic Management

Common medications and substances that can cause nonspecific anxiety symptoms are listed in Table 6.6. Pharmacologic agents used to manage anxiety are listed in Table 6.7.

Antidepressants are effective for treating anxiety, but full benefit may take several weeks, and lower doses are tolerated best. Many clinicians treating anxiety disorders use selective serotonin reuptake inhibitors (SSRIs) as their first choice due to these agents' reliability and effectiveness for panic, generalized anxiety disorders, post-traumatic stress disorder, and obsessive-compulsive disorder. Common side effects are managed with low dose titration; SSRIs have no adjuvant therapeutic effect on pain, unlike serotonin-norepinephrine reuptake inhibitors.[4] Tricyclic antidepressants are effective and inexpensive, and they serve as an adjuvant for neuropathic pain. Tricyclics can promote sleep and appetite but may have a high side-effect burden.

Benzodiazepines are commonly used for the relief of acute anxiety. They have a rapid onset and can reduce nausea, but they are toxic if overdosed

Table 6.4 Summary of Adjustment Stages when Diagnosed with Serious Illness: Pre-Diagnosis and Diagnosis

Pre-Diagnosis	Diagnosis		
Diagnostic process	Phase 1 Initial response	Phase 2 Dysphoria	Phase 3 Adaptation (long-term)
1) Anxiety experience: Normal levels of anxiety and concern Crisis: Psychological and existential	1) Anxiety experience: Disbelief Denial Shock High level of distress, emotions Inability to remember, understand	1) Anxiety experience: Distress ranges: Illness-death Depression, anxiety, insomnia, anorexia Poor concentration Inability to function in daily roles Hope: increased with understanding and awareness of treatment	1) Anxiety experience: Coping strategies: Problem-focused Emotion-focused Meaning-focused
2) Normal adjustment & support: Support systems, personal, religious, spiritual	2) Normal adjustment & support: Compassionate communication skills to deliver bad news	2) Normal adjustment & support: Education and information	2) Normal adjustment & support: Personalized coping styles and strategies
3) Adjustment period: 1 week	3) Adjustment period: Variable, 1–2 weeks	3) Adjustment period: Variable, 1–2 weeks	3) Adjustment period: Variable, 1–2 weeks

From reference 9.

Table 6.5 Summary of Adjustment Stages when Diagnosed with a Serious Illness

Palliative Care	Survivorship
1) Anxiety experience	1) Anxiety experience
Disbelief, denial, shock, crying, withdrawal, isolation, spiritual/religious anger	Greater appreciation, reprioritizing of life values, strengthening of spiritual or religious beliefs
Shift: palliative curing to healing	
2) Normal adjustment & support:	2) Normal adjustment & support:
Palliative care: hope through what is meaningful	National organizations (i.e., programs, tools, resources)
	Physical, emotional well-being support
3) Adjustment period: Weeks	3) Adjustment period: Gradual over many years
From reference 9.	

and can suppress respirations, especially in patients with lung disease, and can cause cognitive impairment.[14] There are risks for abuse and addiction with benzodiazepines, but they are effective in the long term. Use of long-acting agents can prevent the loss of efficacy that can occur with shorter-acting agents.

Antipsychotics are reliable, but long-term use can produce the side effect of movement disorders. This risk makes them a second-line treatment. They are valuable when a rapid anxiolytic effect is needed and if patients cannot tolerate benzodiazepines or have respiratory compromise.[15]

The geriatric population has special considerations, and medication adjustments are required. Treatment of anxiety often reflects the balance between goals and the length of time remaining in life. This is especially true in geriatric palliative care evaluation and treatment. For patients with less than

Table 6.6 Anxiety-Causing Medications and Substances

Alcohol and nicotine withdrawal	Bronchodilators and sympathomimetics
Analgesics	Caffeine (stimulants)
Anticholinergic	Cannabis
Anticonvulsants	Cocaine
Antidepressants	Corticosteroids and anabolic steroids
Antiemetics	Digitalis toxicity
Antihistamines and decongestants	Epinephrine
Antihypertensives	Hallucinogens
Antiparkinsonian drugs	Sedatives (hypnotic withdrawal and paradoxical reaction)
Antipsychotics	
Anesthetics and analgesics	
Benzodiazepines (secondary to initiation and withdrawal)	
From references 1, 4, 5.	

Table 6.7 Common Pharmacologic Treatment Options of Anxiety

Generic Name	Approximate daily dose/ ranges (mg)	Comment
Benzodiazepines		
Alprazolam	0.25–2 tid–qid	Short-acting
Clonazepam	0.5–2 bid–qid	Long-acting
Diazepam	5–10 bid–qid	Long-acting; rapid onset with single PO dosage
Lorazepam	0.5–2 tid–qid	Short-acting; multiple routes, PO, SL, IV, IM, no metabolites
Azapirones		
Buspirone	5–20 tid	Extended time to peak effect similar to antidepressants
Antidepressants		
Serotonin Reuptake Inhibitors		
Citalopram	20–40 daily	New warning from US Food & Drug Administration about doses above 40 mg
Fluoxetine	10–80 daily	Longest half-life among serotonin reuptake inhibitors
Paroxetine	10–60 daily	
Sertraline	50–200 daily	
Tricyclics		
Desipramine	12.5–150 daily	Least sedating tricyclic antidepressant
Imipramine	12.5–150 daily	
Other Antidepressants		
Duloxetine	40–60 daily	
Venlafaxine	75–375 daily	
Mirtazapine	15–60 daily	Promotes sleep and appetite at low doses; oral disintegrating tablets available
Antipsychotics		
Olanzapine	5–15 daily[a]	Oral disintegrating tablets available
Quetiapine	25–200 daily[a]	Preferred for patients with Parkinson's disease
Risperidone	1–3 daily[a]	
Haloperidol	0.5–5 q 2–12h	Inexpensive and multiple routes of administration (IV, PO, and IM)
Antihistamines		
Hydroxyzine	25–50 q 4–6h	Risk of anticholinergic side effects and delirium

[a]In divided doses
From reference 4.

Table 6.8 Nonpharmacologic Anxiety Treatment

Mind-Body Therapy	Posture & Mobility	Touch & Body Work Energetic Therapies	Sense Therapy
Biofeedback	Movement therapy	Massage	Aromatherapy
Psychotherapy	Tai Chi	Reflexology	Music therapy
Guided Imagery	Yoga	Acupressure	Kinesthetics
Hypnosis		Healing Touch	
Meditation		Reiki	
Cognitive Therapy		Therapeutic Touch	
Behavioral Therapy		Polarity Therapy	
Reminiscence/Life Review			
Creating Intention			
Journaling			

From references 17–20.

a few months to live who are minimally ambulatory, benzodiazepines for rapid relief of symptoms or brief treatment can be prescribed. They are considered a second-line drug based on their longer half-life, which causes adverse drug effects. Benzodiazepines overall have a paradoxical effect that may actually cause more anxiety, especially in the elderly, and they are not recommended because they can increase confusion. Typically, tricyclic antidepressants and beta-adrenergic agents are not well tolerated. The most common side effects in the elderly are ataxia, cognitive impairment, and excessive sleepiness. Opioids are indicated for treatment of anxiety secondary to dyspnea in terminally ill patients.[16] Antidepressant therapies are often indicated, and cholinesterase inhibitors may be beneficial.

Nonpharmacologic Treatment

Palliative care includes holistic integrative therapies as well as conventional therapies. Holism and palliative care philosophy are inseparable since they both focus on the total person, with the belief that the mind, body, and spirit are inseparable and interdependent and that health, illness, and dying are manifestations of the life processes of the whole person.[16–21] In both holistic and palliative care, the partnership among the patient, family, and provider generates a sense of empowerment and enables healing (if not necessarily a cure) and transcendence. Nonpharmacologic therapies used for anxiety are outlined in Table 6.8.

Conclusion

Anxiety is a common response in patients and family members and is manifested in various physical, affective, behavioral, and cognitive responses. Palliative care incorporates anxiety in professional practice standards with the goal of anticipating, identifying, assessing, and addressing it via core and interdisciplinary team approaches.

References

1. Dahlin CM. Anxiety, depression and delirium. In: Matzo M, Sherman D., eds. *Palliative Care Nursing: Quality Care to the End of Life*. 4th ed. New York, NY: Springer; 2015:509–39.

2. Thalén-Lindström A, Larsson G, Glimelius B, Johansson B. Anxiety and depression in oncology patients: a longitudinal study of a screening, assessment, and psychosocial support intervention. *Acta Oncol*. 2013; 52(1): 118–27. doi: 10.3109/0284186X.2012.707785.

3. American Psychiatric Association. *Diagnostic and Statistical Manual of Mental Disorders*. 5th ed. Arlington, VA: American Psychiatric Association; 2013. Accessed June 1, 2013, at dsm.psychiatryonline.org.

4. Shuster J. Anxiety. In: Berger A, Shuster J, Von Roenn J., eds. *Palliative Care and Supportive Oncology*. 4th ed. Philadelphia, PA: Lippincott Williams & Wilkins; 2013:552–61.

5. Borneman T, Brown-Saltzman K. Meaning in illness. In: Ferrell B, Coyle N, Paice J, eds. *Oxford Textbook of Palliative Nursing*. 4th ed. New York, NY: Oxford University Press; 2015:554–63.

6. National Comprehensive Cancer Network. NCCN Clinical Practice Guidelines in Oncology (NCCN©). *Distress management* Ver 3.2015. Available at http://www.nccn.org/professionals/physician_gls/pdf/distress.pdf. Accessed October 23, 2016..

7. Brennan J. Adjustment to cancer: coping or personal transition? *Psychooncology*. 2001; 10(1): 1–18.

8. National Cancer Institute. *Adjustment to Cancer: Anxiety and Distress (PDQ®)– Health Professional Version* Available at http://www.cancer.gov/cancertopics/pdq/supportivecare/adjustment/HealthProfessional/page2. Accessed October 23, 2016.

9. National Cancer Institute: PDQ®. *Adjustment to Cancer*. Bethesda, MD: National Cancer Institute. Available at http://cancer.gov/cancertopics/pdq/supportivecare/adjustment/HealthProfessional/page5. Last modified September 15, 2015. Accessed October 23, 2016.

10. Zabora JR. Screening procedures for psychosocial distress. In: Holland JC, Breitbart W, Jacobsen PB, et al., eds. *Psycho-oncology*. New York, NY: Oxford University Press; 2010:653–61.

11. Fineberg L, Houser A. *Assessing family caregiver needs: policy and practice considerations*. Washington DC: AARP Public Policy Institute. Available at http://www.caregiving.org/wp-content/uploads/2010/11/AARP-caregiver-factsheet.pdf. Accessed October 23, 2016.

12. Kutner KS, Kilbourn KM. Bereavement: addressing challenges faced by advanced cancer patients and their caregivers, and their physicians. *Prim Care*. 2009; 36(4): 825–44.

13. Witt-Sherman D, Cheon J. Family caregivers. In: Matzo M, Sherman D, eds. *Palliative Care Nursing: Quality Care to the End of Life*. 4th ed. New York, NY: Springer Publishing; 2015:147–63.

14. Nutt DJ. Overview of diagnosis and drug treatments of anxiety disorders. *CNS Spectr*. 2005; 10(1): 46–59.

15. Ravindran LN, Stein MB. The pharmacologic treatment of anxiety disorders: a review of progress. *J Clin Psychiatry*. 2010; 71: 839–54.

16. Morrison RS, Meier D. *Geriatric Palliative Care*. New York, NY: Oxford University Press; 2014:286–298.

17. Freeman L. *Mosby's Complementary and Alternative Medicine: A Research-Based Approach*. 3rd ed. St. Louis, MO: Mosby Elsevier; 2008.

18. Dossey B, Keengan L, eds. *Holistic Nursing, A Handbook for Practice*. 6th ed. Burlington, MA: Jones and Bartlett Learning; 2013.

19. Snyder M, Lunquist R, eds. *Complementary and Alternative Therapies in Nursing*. New York, NY: Springer; 2010.

20. Matzo M, Sherman D. *Palliative Care Nursing: Quality Care to the End of Life*. 4th ed. New York, NY: Springer; 2010.

21. Quinn J. Transpersonal human caring and healing. In: Dossey B, Keengan L, eds. *Holistic Nursing: A Handbook for Practice*. 6th ed. Burlington, MA: Jones & Bartlett, 2013:107–16.

Chapter 7

Delirium

Peggy S. Burhenn

> **Key Points**
>
> • Delirium is a common, serious medical problem that is underrecognized by healthcare providers. Evidence suggests that frequent assessment of patients can result in increased recognition of delirium, which will allow for earlier intervention.
> • Limited data are available on effective interventions for delirium once it begins; however, proactive prevention strategies have been successful.

Definition

Delirium is defined by the American Psychiatric Association's *Diagnostic and Statistical Manual*, 5th edition (DSM-V) as a disturbance in attention and awareness that develops over a short period of time. It includes an additional cognitive disturbance, and its symptoms are not better explained by another disorder or as a consequence of another medical condition.[1] Delirium is a disturbance in consciousness that has a related change in cognition that occurred over a short period of time (usually hours to days) and is likely caused by a medical condition.[1] A delirium diagnosis requires the presence of an acute onset of or fluctuating course in a change of mental status.

There are three generally recognized subtypes of delirium:[1,2]

• Hyperactive: characterized by a hyperactive level of psychomotor activity, often combined with mood swings, agitation, refusal to cooperate with medical care, hallucinations, and/or inappropriate behavior.[1,2]
• Hypoactive: characterized by a hypoactive level of psychomotor activity that may be accompanied by reduced motor activity, sluggishness, and lethargy that approaches stupor.[1,2]
• Mixed: may have a normal level of psychomotor activity, but attention and awareness are disturbed. Also includes individuals whose activity level rapidly fluctuates between hypoactive and hyperactive.[1,2]

Hyperactive delirium may seem to be most common because its symptoms are more noticeable and disruptive. It has also been associated with medications or drug withdrawal.[1] However, the hypoactive state, often associated with fatigue or lethargy symptoms, is actually more frequent than the hyper-active state but is underdiagnosed.[3]

Pathophysiology

The pathophysiology of delirium is not fully understood. Somatic distur-bances, such as infection, toxins, or metabolic processes, interrupt cen-tral nervous system areas responsible for arousal, perception, and focus.[4] Reduced acetylcholine signaling and excess dopamine signaling, along with elevated pro-inflammatory and anti-inflammatory cytokines, are proposed mechanisms for delirium.[4] Reduced acetylcholinergic signals can directly affect cognition, as witnessed in patients who are administered anticholin-ergic medications (e.g., diphenhydramine, oxybutynin), which can cause confusion.[4] Antidopamine agents given to delirious patients can lessen the symptoms, leading to a theory that excess dopamine plays a role in delirium.[4] Apolipoprotein E epsilon 4 genotype, which is present with an increase in inflammation, was found in a higher percentage of older adults experiencing delirium.[5] Delirium is more likely to be caused by a combination of biological mechanisms than a single cause.[6]

Risk Factors

Development of delirium is multifactorial (Table 7.1).[4,6] Age and pre-existing dementia are the strongest risk factors for developing delirium.[7] Delirium is more common in combination with dementia, and dementia is more likely to

Table 7.1 Factors that Contribute to or Worsen Delirium

Predisposing Factors	Precipitating Factors
Older age (≥75)	Polypharmacy (especially anticholinergic or psychoactive medications)
Dementia	
Previous delirium	Use of urinary catheters
Immobility	Use of restraints
Dehydration	Hypoxia
Malnutrition	Constipation
Visual impairment	Surgery (especially cardiothoracic and vascular)
Hearing impairment	Alcohol excess
Severity of illness	Pain
Comorbidity	Infection
Depression	Frequent environmental changes
History of transient ischemic attack or stroke	Disruption of day/night cycles
Alcohol abuse	Noise and light disturbances

From references 6, 8, 9.

Table 7.2 IWATCHDEATH Mnemonic

I	Infections	Upper respiratory or urinary tract infections, meningitis, sepsis, central nervous system (CNS) abscess
W	Withdrawal	Alcohol or sedatives–hypnotics, barbiturates
A	Acute metabolic conditions	Electrolyte imbalances, hepatic/renal failure, acid–base imbalances
T	Trauma	Head trauma, postoperative, heat stroke, burns
C	CNS pathology	Stroke, CNS metastasis, normal-pressure hydrocephalus, hemorrhage, seizures
H	Hypoxia	Pulmonary or cardiac failure, anemia, pulmonary embolus, carbon monoxide poisoning, hypotension
D	Deficiencies	Vitamin B_{12}, niacin, thiamine, hypovitaminosis
E	Endocrine disorders (sometimes listed as Environmental)	Alteration in diabetes, thyroid, parathyroid, or adrenocortical system, hyperthermia, hypothermia
A	Acute vascular	Encephalopathy, shock, hypertensive emergency
T	Toxins or drugs	Medications, industrial poisons, solvents, pesticides, drugs of abuse, cyanide
H	Heavy metals	Lead, mercury, or manganese

From references 10, 11.

develop after delirium.[6] Age, as an independent factor, may relate to functional age and frailty rather than actual chronological age. Poor functional status, multiple comorbidities, depression, sensory impairment, fluid and electrolyte imbalances, medications, and alcohol can also be associated with increased delirium.[1,7]

Factors that may contribute to or worsen delirium include immobility, dehydration, anticholinergic or psychoactive medication, use of urinary catheters or restraints, hypoxia, malnutrition, constipation, pain, infection, frequent environmental changes, disruption of day–night cycles, noise, and light disturbances (see Table 7.1).[6,10] Serious medical conditions are frequently associated with the development of delirium and the mnemonic IWATCHDEATH was created to outline those medical conditions (Table 7.2).[10]

Assessment

Assessment is essential and includes history, mental and physical examination, and diagnostic. Table 7.3 reviews a comprehensive delirium assessment.

Management

Identification of the cause(s) guides appropriate treatment:
• Manage electrolyte imbalances.
• Reduce medications, especially anticholinergics.

Table 7.3 Delirium Assessment

Delirium Assessment	Description
History	Onset, behavior changes such as agitation or withdrawal, presence of inattention, confusion, hallucination, or alteration in sleep–wake cycle.
Initial assessment	Mental status and cognitive or perceptual disturbances as compared to baseline and use of a delirium tool.
Head-to-toe physical exam	Urinary retention, constipation, or infections in lungs, abdomen, urinary tract, or skin.[11]
Medication review	Anticholinergic drugs, analgesics, benzodiazepines, and hypnotics, among others.[10,11]
Diagnostic testing	Complete blood count; comprehensive metabolic panel, including urea, electrolytes, glucose, calcium, renal function, and liver function
	Serum drug levels depending on medications
	Drug toxicology
	C-reactive protein
	Chest x-ray (review for pneumonia, effusion, and heart abnormalities)
	Blood cultures; pulse oximetry; urinalysis and culture, electrocardiogram[2,4]
	Thyroid function and B12 and folate levels[2]
	Brain imaging (to evaluate for brain metastases), EEG, or abdominal computed tomography for a patient with severe nausea and vomiting and no bowel movements, to rule out an obstruction.[9]
	Oxygen saturation levels (hypoxia) or spinal tap can be done if an infectious process is suspected.

- Treat infections with antibiotics or antifungals.
- Assess for pain and treat it effectively, with scheduled dosing.
- Ensure that eyeglasses and/or hearing aids are in place and working (check batteries).
- Assess for and treat constipation.
- Maintain hydration to prevent dehydration and constipation. Oral route is preferred.
- Ensure oxygenation and prescribe oxygen as necessary.
- Antipsychotics are the drugs of choice for many clinicians. Titrate starting dose and use lower doses for older adults[2] (Table 7.4).
- Institute patient monitoring using a continuous observer or a one-to-one sitter.
- Consider consultation with other disciplines, such as a pharmacist (for medication review), geriatrician, neurologist, psychiatrist, or neuropsychologist who is experienced in cognitive evaluation and treatment.[12]
- Implement nonpharmacologic measures appropriate for the setting.
- Improve orientation to environment and person and ensure continuity of care.

Table 7.4 Pharmacologic Management of Delirium

Class	Agent	Dosing	Comments
Typical antipsychotics	Haloperidol	0.5–2 mg may be given PO, SC, IV, IM q 2–12h. *In older adults:* 0.25–0.5 mg PO q 4h or 1–2 mg IM up to q 2h (maximum dose 5 mg/day)	Increased rates of extrapyramidal side effects in higher doses (4.5 mg/day or above). Risk of QT prolongation: monitor ECG at baseline and daily, especially with IV and higher doses. Maintain normal serum potassium and magnesium levels. IM absorption may be poor. IV route not FDA approved. May precipitate with heparin; 2-mL saline flush is recommended prior to IV administration.
	Chlorpromazine	12.5–50 mg q 4–6h PO, IV, IM, PR, SC	Higher level of anticholinergic and sedating effects than haloperidol. Monitor in intensive care setting.
Atypical antipsychotics (alternative if intolerant to haloperidol, fewer extrapyramidal side effects)	Olanzapine	2.5–5 mg q 12–24h PO, ODT, IM	Poorer response in older adults, those with pre-existing dementia, and hypoactive delirium. May cause sedation.
	Risperidone	0.25–1 mg q 12–24h PO, ODT	Monitor for orthostatic hypotension and extrapyramidal side effects in higher doses.
	Aripiprazole	5–30 mg q 24h PO or IM	May be more effective in hypoactive delirium.
	Quetiapine	12.5–100 mg q 12–24h PO	Monitor for orthostatic hypotension. May cause sedation.

No agents are approved by the US Food & Drug Administration (FDA) for use in delirium. Dose recommendations vary by source. Typical and atypical antipsychotics carry an FDA warning of increased mortality in elderly patients with dementia-related psychosis.

ODT, oral disintegrating tablets.

From references 2, 8, 10, 13, 14.

- Limit staffing changes to foster familiarity.
- Encourage mobility and engagement in social activities. Promote sleep–wake cycle with appropriate daytime light and sleep hygiene measures. Reduce noise and minimize sleep interruptions by avoiding nighttime nursing or medical interventions.
- Involve patient and family in care through visits and familiar items from home.
- Avoid additional trauma or complications (e.g., eliminate urinary catheters by promoting regular toileting, prevent pressure injury by regularly assessing skin using valid assessment scales, provide adequate nutritional intake by offering nutritional supplements and finger food, limit transfer to other units, avoid restraints).
- Provide support and counseling to patients and family. Delirium is common at the end-of-life and can be a prognostic indicator of impending death.

Pharmacology

Currently, there are no approved drugs to treat delirium. Sedatives and antipsychotics are often used with the following guidelines:

- Keep the use of sedatives to a minimum. Consider the benefits and burdens of one medication over another.
- Use one drug at a time. Start at the lowest dose and increase as necessary after 2 hours.
- Review all medications at least every 24 hours.
- While titrating drugs, provide one-on-one care.

When drug therapy is required, haloperidol has been the gold standard but may cause extrapyramidal side effects.[13]

Conclusion

Delirium is a distressing experience for patients, caregivers, and healthcare professionals alike. Although the evidence for effective delirium interventions is limited, systematic assessment and modification of risk factors appear to be an effective approach.

References

1. American Psychiatric Association. Delirium. In: *Diagnostic and Statistical Manual of Mental Disorders*. 5th ed. Arlington, VA, American Psychiatric Association; 2013:596–602.
2. British Geriatrics Society. *Guidelines for the prevention, diagnosis and management of delirium in older people in hospital*. 2006. Available at http://www.bgs.org.uk/index.php/clinicalguides/170-clinguidedeliriumtreatment%3Fshowall%3D%26limitstart%3D. Accessed October 23, 2016.

3. Hosie A, Davidson PM, Agar M, et al. Delirium prevalence, incidence, and implications for screening in specialist palliative care inpatient settings: a systematic review. *Palliat Med*. 2013; 27: 486–98.

4. Krishnan V, Leung LY, Caplan LR. A neurologist's approach to delirium: diagnosis and management of toxic metabolic encephalopathies. *Eur J Intern Med*. 2014; 25: 112–6.

5. van Munster BC, Korevaar JC, Zwinderman AH, et al. The association between delirium and the apolipoprotein E epsilon 4 allele: new study results and a meta-analysis. *Am J Geriatr Psychiatry*. 2009; 17: 856–62.

6. Inouye SK, Westendorp RG, Saczynski JS. Delirium in elderly people. *Lancet*. 2014; 383: 911–22.

7. Tullmann D, Fletcher K, Foreman M. Delirium. In: Boltz M, ed. *Evidence-Based Geriatric Nursing Protocols for Best Practice*. 4th ed. New York, NY: Springer; 2012:186–199.

8. Gershon K. In: Dahlin C, Lynch M, eds. *Core Curriculum for the Advanced Practice Hospice and Palliative Registered Nurse, Delirium*. 2nd ed. Pittsburgh, PA: Hospice and Palliative Nurses Association; 2013.

9. Whitlock EL, Torres BA, Lin N, et al. Postoperative delirium in a substudy of cardiothoracic surgical patients in the BAG-RECALL clinical trial. *Anesth Analg*. 2014; 118: 809–17.

10. Caplan JP, Cassem NH, Murray GB, Park JM, Stern TA. Delirious patients. In: Stern TA, Fricchione GL, Cassem NH, Jellinek MS, Rosenbaum JF, eds. *Massachuetts General Hospital Handbook of General Hospital Psychiatry*. 6th ed. Philadelphia, PA: Saunders Elsevier; 2010:93–104.

11. Gower LE, Gatewood MO, Kang CS. Emergency department management of delirium in the elderly. *West J Emerg Med*. 2012; 13: 194–201.

12. National Comprehensive Cancer Network. *Senior Adult Oncology Guideline*. 2016. Available at https://www.nccn.org/professionals/physician_gls/pdf/senior.pdf. Accessed October 23, 2016.

13. Breitbart W, Alici Y. Evidence-based treatment of delirium in patients with cancer. *J Clin Oncol*. 2012; 30: 1206–14.

14. National Comprehensive Cancer Network. *Palliative Care*. 2016. Available at https://www.nccn.org/professionals/physician_gls/pdf/palliative.pdf. Accessed October 23, 2016,

Chapter 8

Depression and Suicide

John D. Chovan

Key Points

- Although a depressed mood is a natural response of patients and their families to a diagnosis of, being treated for, living with, and dying from a chronic, life-threatening illness, depression can lead to thoughts and actions of self-harm that can result in death.
- The grief response, before or after the death of a loved one, does not follow a well-defined linear path but is a journey that is personal to each individual. If not resolved, it can manifest in depressive symptoms.

Definition of Depression

The term *depression* has a technical definition but is often used colloquially in healthcare. When a person says, "I'm depressed," it does not necessarily mean the person has assessed and diagnosed himself or herself according to evidence-based standards. It often means that they are feeling blue, have low spirits, or are unhappy. It may also mean that they are lonely, having physical or psychic pain, or are angry and need to talk. Motivating a person to the point of being able to report "I'm depressed" may be a very complex challenge. For clarity, the terms used in this chapter are:

Mood: The state of one's emotions at a particular point in time[1]

Sadness: The feeling of being in low spirits or being unhappy, also called a depressed mood.[1] The World Health Organization defines depressed mood as "a low mood that may be expressed in a number of ways— sadness, misery, low spirits, inability to enjoy anything, gloom, rejection, feeling blue. ... It becomes pathological when it is persistent, pervasive, unresponsive, painful, or out of proportion to the individual's life circumstances."[2(pp. 17–18)]

Depressive symptoms: The behavioral indicators associated with a depressed mood. These are described in detail later and include sleep changes, anhedonia, guilt, helplessness, hopelessness, changes in energy level, reduced ability to concentrate, appetite changes, psychomotor slowing, and suicidal ideation or attempts.[1] Depressive symptoms can worsen over time in frequency, severity, duration, and impact on functioning to the point of causing disability, thus meeting criteria for a depressive disorder.[3]

Depressive episode: A pathological state that meets predefined criteria based on the existence of a depressed mood or anhedonia as well as five of nine particular depressive symptoms for at least 2 weeks. Most encounters in palliative care and hospice in which the patient says "I'm depressed" will present a constellation of symptoms that very likely do not meet the criteria for a depressive episode.[4]

Depressive disorder: One of the constellation of pathological mood syndromes in which the hallmark feature is severe and persistent depressed mood and associated pathology, limiting one's ability to function in social, occupational, or other important settings. These include major depressive disorder, pervasive depressive disorder, premenstrual dysphoric disorder, substance-induced depression, and depression due to another medical condition. Some palliative care and hospice patients will have a chronic, life-threatening somatic illness in addition to a depressive disorder.[4]

To provide optimal care, the palliative advanced practice registered nurse (APRN) must understand the symptomatology of both somatic and psychiatric illness and the interplay between them.

Depressed Mood and Life-Threatening Illness

Throughout the course of a chronic, life-threatening illness, a patient's response to the illness is often a waxing and waning mood. Patients and their families are often faced with very difficult decisions that can trigger depressive symptoms and thoughts of suicide. As a member of the interdisciplinary team, the APRN assesses for, and plans interventions to alleviate these symptoms.[3-5]

Epidemiology of Depression in Chronic Illness

Depression can occur in many conditions and illnesses, with some conditions having a higher rate of depression (Table 8.1).

History and Pathology

When a person reports experiencing depressive symptoms, the APRN should consider reversible physical causes of the symptoms (Box 8.1).[1] For example, hypothyroidism causes symptoms that mimic depression and can be corrected medically, often with levothyroxine (Synthroid). It can be detected with a blood test that measures circulating levels of thyroid-stimulating hormone (TSH) and thyroxine (T_4). Metastatic disease to the brain can cause mood swings, including depression, as the lesions alter function in mood-related foci of the cerebrum. Normal-pressure hydrocephalus can cause gait and mood changes that mimic depressive symptoms; a consult

Table 8.1 Depression in Chronic Illness

Chronic Illness	% Experiencing Depression
Myocardial infarction	40–65
Parkinson's disease	40
Multiple sclerosis	40
Chronic pain syndrome	30–54
Cancer	25
Diabetes	25
Coronary artery disease	18–20
Stroke	10–27

Adapted from WebMD. Dealing with Chronic Illness and Dperession 2016. http://www.webmd.com/depression/guide/chronic-illnesses-depression#1
Accessed October 23, 2016

to neurology or neuropsychiatry would be appropriate. Unmanaged pain is a common cause of stress, and subsequently somatic symptoms and depressive symptoms, yet it is correctible. Pain can include distress from insomnia, anorexia, dysphagia, and existential rumination, which can lead the patient to ask, "Why me?" Appropriate total pain management can alleviate these stressors and their comorbid depressive symptoms. If potential physiological causes are ruled out, or detected and treated, but the symptoms remain, the APRN can conclude that the symptoms are psychiatric and not due to a correctible physical cause.

The process of taking a history allows the palliative APRN to build rapport with the patient and family when evaluating a new patient for depressive symptoms. Onset, duration, measures that exacerbate it or alleviate it, and amount of debility that the symptoms induce are all features that give insight into how to approach treatment. The therapeutic use of self allows the APRN to defuse any anxiety or reticence about discussing depression, particularly if the distress is in any way related to fear of rejection and the stigma of mental illness.

Box 8.1 Physical Causes of Depression

Brain tumors
Cardiac surgery
Hypothyroidism
Hypoxia
Obstructive sleep apnea
Postpartum
Seizures
Strokes
Traumatic brain injury
From reference 1.

Monoamine therapy, such as the monoamine oxidase inhibitors (MAOIs; e.g., phenelzine [Nardil]), tricyclic antidepressants (TCAs; e.g., amitriptyline [Elavil]), selective serotonin reuptake inhibitors (SSRIs; e.g., citalopram [Celexa]), and serotonin–norepinephrine reuptake inhibitors (SNRIs; e.g., venlafaxine [Effexor]) do offer symptomatic relief. With these therapies, there is often a protracted delay between therapy initiation and onset of symptom relief. Their effect on depressive symptoms is inconsistent. When symptoms are detected before permanent neurological changes take effect, the symptoms can be reversed, and treatment eventually can be discontinued. More severe symptoms, however, will require life-long treatment.[6]

Assessment

A focused history and physical examination will determine the need for appropriate diagnostic tests and their interpretation. The palliative APRN should review the patient's history and record for prior history of depression. If the patient has a history of depression, the APRN should find out what treatments were initiated and their effectiveness. The APRN should also inquire about other mental health issues, including bipolar disorder, personality disorders, disorders that emerge in childhood, and schizophrenia. The APRN must be aware of physiological conditions that can contribute to or mimic depression. The family history should examine the patient's and family's history of suicide. Exposure to a suicide or suicide attempt is a major risk factor for suicide. A medication history should help determine interventions for depression. It should include specific medications that were helpful in the past and those that were not and any allergies to medications or products in pharmaceuticals. The medication review should include all current prescription medication, over-the-counter preparations, supplements, and allergies in order to avoid known sensitivities and to reduce the risk of drug–drug interactions.[7] Finally, there should be discussion about the patient's and the family's knowledge and beliefs about psychiatric illness, pharmacotherapy, and complementary and alternative therapies. The reader is referred to The Textbook of Palliative Nursing, chapter 4, Assessing Patients and Families,[7] for detailed information.

All persons with chronic illness are at risk for depression.[8] Other risk factors for depression are listed in Table 8.2. The physical exam should be focused on mood and psychomotor changes and should include the following:[4]

Depressed mood: A depressed mood is characterized by negative emotions as reported by the patient. Simply asking "How is your mood?" can elicit a response from the patient that indicates an unaltered mood (euthymia) or a mood that is not normal for him or her (dysthymia). "Is this a change from your usual mood?" will help distinguish the patient's current state from his or her baseline and will give insight into the duration of a possible depressive episode.

Sleep changes: Decreased need for sleep, early morning wakening, or an increased need for sleep can all indicate depression. Questions can

Table 8.2 Risk Factors for Depression and Suicide in Adults

Domain	Risk Factor	At Risk for Depression	At Risk for Suicide
Mood	Depressed mood	Depression as a child or teen	Feel hopeless, socially isolated, or lonely
Stressors	Stressful life event • Loss • Illness • Military service • Financial/legal problems	Yes	Yes
Substance abuse	Abuse of alcohol, illegal drugs, and/or prescription drugs	Yes	Yes; can worsen thoughts of suicide and can instill recklessness or impulsivity enough to act on thoughts
Family	Genetic link or environmental exposure to mental illness, substance abuse, or suicide	Blood relatives	Family history History of violence and abuse including physical, emotional, and/or sexual abuse
Psychiatric	Any psychiatric disorder but especially anxiety, post-traumatic stress disorder, personality disorders	Yes; In addition to: • Borderline personality disorder • Certain personality traits, such as having low self-esteem and being overly dependent, self-critical, or pessimistic	Yes; In addition to: • Psychosis • Paranoia
Somatic illness	Chronic or life-threatening illness; pain	Yes	Yes
Medications		Regimen of certain medications, such as some high blood pressure medications or sleeping pills	Initiation of an antidepressant for symptoms of depression
Development			Identification as bisexual, homosexual, or transgender with an unsupportive family or in a hostile environment. In adolescents and children, being unsure of sexual orientation
Means			Access to firearms
History of suicide			Previous suicide attempt

Adapted from. Haggerty J. Risk Factors for Depression http://psychcentral.com/lib/risk-factors-for-depression/ Pysch Central Accessed October 23, 2016.

include: "How are you sleeping? Any difficulty falling asleep? Once you fall asleep, do you stay asleep? Once you wake up in the middle of the night, do you have trouble falling asleep? Do you sleep until your planned waking time? Has this changed from your usual sleep schedule?" Changes in sleep patterns are associated with depression, particularly sleep difficulties in the early to the middle part of the sleep cycle.

Lack of interests or anhedonia: The depressed patient may report lack of interest in activities he or she used to enjoy or a general lack of interest in anything. The APRN might ask, "What sorts of activities are you interested in doing? Has this interest changed recently?"

Beck's Cognitive Triad: Aaron Beck described changes in thinking about the self, the world, and the future as indicators of depression.[9] Excessive guilt and feelings of worthlessness indicate thoughts about the self and can be elicited by asking the patient, "Tell me about your feelings of self-worth. Are there things you feel guilty about?" Thinking about the world is captured by asking the patient to describe how others view him or her from their perspective. "Are you feeling helpless and that others do not want to help you?" And, finally, the patient may see the future as dim when depressed and may believe that there is no way out of his or her current situation: "Do you feel hopeless?"

Energy: Changes in level of energy, typically decreases, are associated with depression: "How's your energy level?"

Concentration: Changes in ability to concentrate, typically more difficulty concentrating, are associated with depression: "How is your ability to concentrate?"

Appetite: Changes in appetite, either up or down, and significant weight loss without intentional dieting are features associated with depression. The APRN can ask, "How is your appetite? Is that a change from your usual appetite? Have you lost weight? How much? Over what period of time?"

Psychomotor slowing: Moving more slowly than usual; difficulty initiating activity, such as getting out of bed or off the couch; slower gait; and slower speech are symptoms of depression. Self-report is not as reliable as observation by a friend or family member. The APRN can ask the patient whether the friend or family member has mentioned anything unusual about the patient's ability to move or walk.

Suicidal thoughts or attempts are associated with depression. Risk factors for suicide include exposure to a completed suicide or suicide attempt, thoughts about committing suicide, planning to commit suicide, possessing the means to commit suicide, having access to the means to commit suicide, the potential lethality of the means (e.g., the amount of physical damage that the means could cause), and an unsuccessful attempt at suicide in the past. Other risk factors for suicide are listed in Table 8.2. The APRN should screen for suicide by asking these questions:

1. Has anyone close to you attempted or completed suicide?
2. Have you ever tried to hurt yourself?
3. Are you currently thinking about hurting yourself?
4. Do you have a plan?

5. How are you planning on doing it?
6. Do you have the means to implement such a plan?

A mnemonic for the features of depression is SIG E CAPS, a play on the prescription to "Take (Sig) energy (E) capsules (Caps)," which stands for **S**leep changes, **I**nterest changes, **G**uilt or hopelessness, **E**nergy decreases, **C**oncentration difficulties, **A**ppetite changes, **P**sychomotor changes, **S**uicidal ideation[10].

If the patient or family member reports that the patient has thoughts about committing suicide, along with a plan and access to the means, safety becomes paramount. The palliative APRN should make a safety contract with the patient if possible and then call for assistance from mental health colleagues to have the patient transferred to a setting with more advanced psychiatric help.[1,11,12]

When someone takes his or her own life, the first question typically asked is, "Why?" Even when a suicide note is left behind, questions remain unanswered. Suicide can trigger physical or psychiatric illness in the surviving members of the family and friends. The palliative APRN will be better able to support the survivors if he or she has thought about his or her own beliefs and attitudes about suicide and how it fits into his or her own philosophy of life. Exploring other people's views, including other members of the transdisciplinary team, is beneficial. It allows the APRN to anticipate his or her own personal reactions and perspectives so he or she can best help members of the patient's family and other team members.

Ongoing Assessment

At the initial encounter, the palliative APRN collects baseline data. At subsequent encounters, the APRN assesses the patient and family for any changes from this baseline, using them to measure progress, emerging issues, and the effectiveness of treatments: "Compared to [before or last time] we met, is it the same, better, or worse?"[7] During each encounter, the palliative APRN builds a trusting relationship with the patient and family to facilitate the sharing of information.[1] This is particularly important when discussing mental health issues because of the sensitive nature of mental illness and the stigma associated with it. The palliative APRN continues to build the database from which an appropriate plan of care will be derived, including evidence of risk for and symptoms of depression, as well as related substance abuse and risk for suicide. The acuity of each symptom is also determined:[3] frequency (e.g., nearly every day, most days, 2 or 3 days per week, weekly, once per month or less), duration (e.g., nonstop, months, days, just that day, a few hours), and impact on daily function (e.g., can or cannot work, can or cannot take care of one's own needs, can or cannot cook for oneself, bedbound).

Differential Diagnosis

The differential diagnosis for depressive symptoms is shown in Table 8.3.[4] When these symptoms are observed, the palliative APRN collects appropriate

CHAPTER 8 Depression and Suicide

Table 8.3 Differential Diagnosis for Depression

Differential	Description	Comments
Grief	Normal emotional reaction to a loss. Over time, can evolve into a depressive disorder.	The prominent symptom is emptiness, not anhedonia and depressed mood. Self-esteem is preserved, although feelings of sadness come and go. Persons experiencing grief may express a desire to be with the lost loved one, but they do not think of suicide as a way to make the bad feelings go away.
Depressed mood	Sadness or feeling blue	A depressed mood by itself is not a depressive disorder but rather a stand-alone symptom; however, it can be debilitating.
Adjustment disorder	Clinical disorder as defined in DSM-V. Difficulty adapting to a new sense of normal.	The parameters for depressive symptoms (number, severity, duration, and impact) are of a lesser degree and do not meet the criteria for major depressive disorder.
Major depressive disorder	A depressive disorder characterized in DSM-V by multiple symptoms over an extended period of time.	Five or more symptoms (SIG E CAPS: Sleep changes, Interest changes, Guilt or hopelessness, Energy decreases, Concentration difficulties, Appetite changes, Psychomotor changes, Suicidal ideation), including depressed mood, for at least 2 weeks. May be recurrent.
Bipolar disorder	A mood disorder characterized by alternating depression and manic mood states.	Must meet criteria for major depression during depressive episodes and either mania or hypomania as defined in DSM-V (DIG FAST: Distractibility, Irresponsibility, Grandiosity, Flight of ideas, Activity increases, Sleep is decreased, Talkative)

From reference 4.

data to differentiate subpathological conditions, such as normal grief, from higher-acuity conditions based on the constellation of signs and symptoms, their characteristics, and the impact on the individual and family.

Management and Interventional Techniques

Evidence-based interventions and approaches for helping patients with depressive symptoms are based on the following principles: (1) the patient–clinician relationship is important to the development of a successful plan of care, (2) the patient and the family are at the center of the therapeutic relationship, and (3) an interdisciplinary approach will result in optimal care. Ongoing monitoring of effectiveness is key to managing depression.[1]

Psychotherapy

Current evidence for depression shows that management is best when it includes psychotherapy as well as pharmacologic management. For patients and families with depressive symptoms, processing their feelings aloud can help them find peace, make meaning out of their situation, and develop hope. The challenge for patients with serious illness is finding a supportive and affordable group therapy or therapists at a convenient location. The palliative APRN with training in therapy provides opportunities for the person to process his or her feelings. Otherwise, a referral to a professional trained in brief therapy, cognitive-behavioral therapy, or other therapeutic techniques can be made to manage depressive symptoms in palliative settings.[13,14]

Pharmacologic Management

Pharmaceutical therapy is the most common technique used for managing depressive symptoms. This choice, however, may depend on the patient's prognosis. For patients who have a prognosis of longer than 2–3 months, there are more options. SSRIs and SNRIs are first-line medications for treating depressive symptoms.[6] Table 8.4 lists the generic and brand names of commonly prescribed antidepressants. Table 8.5 lists the side effects of SSRIs and SNRIs.

A common patient concern is the sexual side effects of the SSRIs, specifically orgasmic delay in men and women and erectile dysfunction in men. These side effects can be treated with psychotherapy or with the addition of bupropion (Wellbutrin). Typically, SSRIs and SNRIs are given only after other antidepressants, if any, have been given sufficient time to wash out of the body. Like any other medication in palliative care, the drug is initiated at the lowest therapeutic dose and the dosage is adjusted as needed. Subtherapeutic effects are often observed in the first few weeks, but full therapeutic effect is achieved in 6–8 weeks after pharmacotherapy has started. Citalopram (Celexa) and its levoisomer escitalopram (Lexapro) have been used to control depressive symptoms while minimizing side effects. Duloxetine (Cymbalta) is used to alleviate depressive symptoms and some somatic symptoms of depression. Mirtazapine (Remeron) has been shown to have a more rapid onset than SSRIs when used to treat major depression,

Table 8.4 Common Pharmacotherapies for Depression

Class	Generic Name	Brand Name
Selective serotonin reuptake inhibitors (SSRIs)	citalopram	Celexa
	escitalopram	Lexapro
	fluoxetine	Prozac
	paroxetine	Paxil
	sertraline	Zoloft
	vilazodone	Viibryd
Serotonin–norepinephrine reuptake inhibitors (SNRIs)	desvenlafaxine	Pristiq
	duloxetine	Cymbalta
	venlafaxine	Effexor
Other Antidepressants		
Serotonin & dopamine reuptake inhibitor	bupropion	Wellbutrin
Serotonin & catecholamine reuptake inhibitor	mirtazapine	Remeron

From reference 6.

but the side-effect profile is often debilitating.[15] Off-label uses of mirtazapine include treating anxiety symptoms, nausea, pruritus, insomnia, and anorexia. When either discontinuing a medication or switching to a new medication, a taper or cross-taper over 2 weeks is required to avoid discontinuation effects.[6]

Current evidence shows that, for moderate to severe depression, symptoms are better controlled by a combination of talk therapy and medication than by either modality alone. But mild to moderate depression has

Table 8.5 Common Side Effects of SSRIs and SNRIs

SSRIs	SNRIs
Agitation	Agitation
Anorexia	Discontinuation syndrome
Anxiety	Headache
Constipation	Hypertension (dose-related)
Diarrhea	Nausea
Discontinuation syndrome	Sleep disturbances
Dizziness	Sweating
Dry mouth	Tremor
Headache	
Insomnia	
Nausea	
Sexual dysfunction	
Somnolence	
Sweating	
Tremor	

From reference 6.

been shown to respond equally well to pharmacotherapy, to talk therapy, or both.[13] Referral to a mental health specialist is essential for patients with severe depression.[16]

Complex Medication Use

The SSRIs and SNRIs that are used today are third- and fourth-generation medications that manipulate the monoamine neurotransmitters. Earlier medications with similar effects are the MAOIs and the TCAs. If a patient is taking a drug from one of these classes, the palliative APRN needs to be aware of the patient's risk for a life-threatening condition—serotonin syndrome (SS) (Box 8.2). Of note, one substance commonly taken by patients is St. John's wort, an over-the-counter herbal medication that is used to augment mood and to treat other ailments by increasing serotonin levels. Although not approved by the US Food and Drug Administration as a pharmaceutical, St. John's wort, in combination with other serotonergic drugs, can cause SS.[17]

MAOIs and TCAs must not be taken with SSRIs and SNRIs. If the patient's depressive symptoms become refractory to his or her older medications, then a washout period of 2 weeks is required before starting the more current medications. If the patient is taking an MAOI, diet must be restricted to avoid foods high in tyramine, a precursor to serotonin. These foods include some cheeses; beer; dried meats, such as salami and pepperoni; chicken livers; meat bouillons and gravies; and fermented foods, such as kimchi, sauerkraut, tofu, soy sauce, and fish sauce.[18]

Management of Concomitant Diagnoses

Some bipolar disorders are characterized by the existence of a depressed mood and are treated with mood stabilizers. The use of an SSRI or SNRI in a patient with bipolar disorder may trigger a manic episode, a pathological state that may have been revealed in the history. If mania is discovered, SSRI and SNRI antidepressants should be avoided. In these cases, mood elevators (e.g., lithium) are the first-line therapy.[1]

Box 8.2 Serotonin Syndrome: A Life-Threatening Condition

Sustained levels of serotonin in the synaptic cleft alleviate depressive symptoms. Combinations of medications that increase the level of serotonin in the synaptic cleft, however, can be additive and cause concentrations of serotonin to rise to dangerously high levels. When this happens, evidence of serotonin syndrome (SS) emerges.

SS presents as three or more of the following symptoms: agitation; diarrhea; heavy sweating not due to activity; fever; mental status changes, such as confusion or hypomania; muscle spasms (myoclonus); overactive reflexes (hyperreflexia); shivering; tremor; and uncoordinated movements (ataxia).

This is a crisis situation that is typically treated by stopping the medication and administering benzodiazepines, intravenous fluids, and cyproheptadine, a serotonin antagonist antihistamine.[6]

Depression can also be accompanied by psychosis, or not being in touch with reality. If psychotic features are also present, the patient requires antipsychotics in addition to antidepressants. These medications can cause metabolic changes (such as hyperlipidemia, hyperglycemia, and prolonged QTc interval) that can precipitate other comorbid conditions. For example, some antipsychotics cause hyperlipidemia, which can lead to coronary artery disease and distributed atherosclerosis. Hyperglycemia can lead to diabetes mellitus. Cardiac conduction can be affected, such as a prolonged QTc interval, leaving the patient at risk for lethal dysrhythmias. Any side effects should be treated according to evidence-based guidelines. Of note, the palliative APRN should use caution when attempting to manage agitation or delirium in a patient who is already taking antipsychotics as the patient's illness proceeds toward end-of-life. High levels of antipsychotics can lead to neuroleptic malignant syndrome (NMS), a life-threatening emergency characterized by muscle cramps and tremors, fever, symptoms of autonomic nervous system instability like unstable blood pressure, and alterations in mental status (agitation, delirium, or coma). NMS is treated symptomatically, with ice packs for fever, supportive respiratory and circulatory care, and dantrolene for muscle rigidity.[6]

SS and NMS are life-threatening emergencies that must be treated emergently. NMS is distinguished from SS by the presence of bradykinesia, muscle rigidity, and elevated white blood cell count and plasma creatine kinase level. Prevention of these conditions should include a referral to a mental health professional for alternative approaches to optimal patient care.[1,6]

Safe Prescribing

Safe prescribing begins with a thorough history of the patient that includes diet, allergies, and medications, both historical and current, and herbal supplements. Avoiding concomitant substances (such as St. John's wort) and foods that induce serotonin will decrease the likelihood of SS. Understanding the patient's use of antipsychotics and safe prescribing will help avoid NMS.

Safe prescribing also includes minimizing the availability of lethal doses of any medication that could be used as a means of suicide. For example, consider a patient who has depressive symptoms and is being treated for anxiety with benzodiazepines. The patient has a 30-day supply of lorazepam (Ativan) in 10 mg tablets. In a moment of despair due to new-onset depression, this patient could kill himself by taking all 30 pills at once: the maximum safe dosage of lorazepam in 24 hours is 10 mg.[19] Even acetaminophen in large enough quantities can damage an otherwise healthy liver and cause death.[20] A patient who is planning suicide could hoard pills over time to build a lethal stash. The palliative APRN should consider dosages, amounts, and refills of medication to prevent their lethal use. Interventions and therapy relieve some symptoms, so the patient may be less fatigued and more energetic while still being at risk for suicide. The palliative APRN must remain vigilant for depression and assess for suicidal ideation, plan, means, and access at every interaction. The challenge is tailoring such practices to promote a supportive encounter that meets the needs of the patient without enabling a dysfunctional response.[1]

Nonpharmacologic Interventions

Depressive symptoms can be co-managed with physical activity, such as walking, swimming, and yoga, and with proper nutrition.[21,22] Talk therapies can assist patients and families to find a new sense of normal and to create meaning in the patient's situation, which can mitigate depressive symptoms.[1] Other modalities, such as meditation, prayer, guided imagery, music therapy, aromatherapy, and acupuncture, have been shown to alleviate depressive symptoms.[23]

Conclusion

Symptoms of depression are very common in patients diagnosed with serious illness, advanced illness, progressive chronic illness, life-limiting illness, and their families. Disentangling the causes for the constellation of depression symptoms requires keen insights and a strong base of scientific knowledge. Helping patients to cope emotionally maximizes their quality of life, the ultimate goal of palliative care.

References

1. American Psychiatric Association. *Practice Guideline for Treatment of Patients with Major Depressive Disorder.* 3rd ed. Arlington, VA: American Psychiatric Association; 2010. Available at https://psychiatryonline.org/pb/assets/raw/sitewide/practice_guidelines/guidelines/mdd.pdf. Accessed October 23, 2016.

2. Isaac M, Janca A, Sartorius N, eds. *ICD-10 Symptom Glossary for Mental Disorders.* Geneva, Switzerland: World Health Organization; 1994.

3. Porche K, Reymond L, Callaghan JO, Charles M. Depression in palliative care patients: a survey of assessment and treatment practices of Australian and New Zealand palliative care specialists. *Aust Health Rev.* 2014; 38(1): 44–50.

4. American Psychiatric Association. *Diagnostic and Statistical Manual of Mental Disorders.* 5th ed. Arlington, VA: American Psychiatric Association; 2013.

5. Lloyd-Williams M, Payne S, Reeve J, Dona RK. Thoughts of self-harm and depression as prognostic factors in palliative care patients. *J Affect Disord.* 2014; 166(Sep): 324–9.

6. Stahl SM. *Essential Psychopharmacology: The Prescriber's Guide.* 4th ed. New York, NY: Cambridge University Press; 2013.

7. Chovan JD, Cluxton D, Rancour P. Assessing patients and families. In: Ferrell B, Coyle N, Paice J, eds. *Textbook of Palliative Nursing.* 4th ed. New York, NY: Oxford University Press; 2015.

8. American Psychological Association. *Coping with a Diagnosis of Chronic Illness.* Psychology Help Center. Available at http://www.apa.org/helpcenter/chronic-illness.aspx. Updated August, 2013. Accessed October 23, 2016.

9. Gotlib IH, Hammen CL, eds. *Handbook of Depression.* 3rd ed. New York, NY: Guildford; 2014.

10. Gross, C. (1998). SIGECAPS. *Psychiatry Resident Manual.* Boston, MA: Massachusetts General Hospital.

11. Mayo Clinic. *Suicide and Suicidal Thoughts*. Diseases and Conditions. Available at http://www.mayoclinic.org/diseases-conditions/suicide/basics/definition/con-20033954. Published August 2015. Accessed October 23, 2016.

12. Trevino KM, Abbott CH, Fisch MJ, Friedlander RJ, Duberstein PR, Prigerson HG. Patient–oncologist alliance as protection against suicidal ideation in young adults with advanced cancer. *Cancer*. 2014; 120(15): 2272–81.

13. Okumura Y, Ichikura K. Efficacy and acceptability of group cognitive behavioral therapy for depression: a systematic review and meta-analysis. *J Affect Disord*. 2014; 164(Aug): 155–64.

14. Li M, Fitzgerald P, Rodin G. Evidence-based treatment of depression in patients with cancer. *J Clin Oncol*. 2013; 31(28): 3612.

15. Watanabe N, Omori IM, Nakagawa A, et al. Mirtazapine versus other antidepressive agents for depression. *Cochrane Database Syst Rev*. 2011, Issue 12. Art. No.: CD006528.

16. Rayner L, Price A, Hotopf M, Higginson IJ. The development of evidence-based European guidelines on the management of depression in palliative cancer care. *Eur J Cancer*. 2011; 47(5): 702–12.

17. Davis SA, Feldman SR, Taylor SL. Use of St. John's wort in potentially dangerous combinations. *J Altern Complement Med*. 2014; 20(7): 578–9.

18. Holden KJ. *Meal Ideas and Menus: Avoiding High-Tyramine Foods Made Easy*. North Wales, PA: Teva Neuroscience, Inc.; 2006.

19. U.S. Food & Drug Administration. *Ativan (lorazepam) tablets*. FDA Drug Label. Available at http://www.accessdata.fda.gov/drugsatfda_docs/label/2007/017794s034s035lbl.pdf. Accessed October 23, 2016.

20. U.S. Food & Drug Administration. *FDA Drug Safety Communication: Prescription Acetaminophen Products to be Limited to 325 mg Per Dosage Unit; Boxed Warning Will Highlight Potential for Severe Liver Failure*. Drug Safety and Availability. Available at http://www.fda.gov/drugs/drugsafety/ucm239821.htm#aihp. Accessed October 23, 2016.

21. Danielsson L, Papoulias I, Petersson E-L, Carlsson J, Waern M. Exercise or basic body awareness therapy as add-on treatment for major depression: a controlled study. *J Affect Disord*. 2014; 168(Oct): 98–106.

22. O'Neil A, Quirk SE, Housed S, et al. Relationship between diet and mental health in children and adolescents: a systematic review. *Am J Public Health*. 2014; 104(10): e31–42.

23. Purohit MP, Wells RE, Zafonte RD, Davis RB, Phillips RS. Neuropsychiatric symptoms and the use of complementary and alternative medicine. *PM R*. 2013; 5(1): 24–31.

Chapter 9

Palliative Emergencies

Marcia J. Buckley and Ann Syrett

Key Points

- Hemorrhage is a frightening experience for both patient and family. The palliative advanced practice registered nurse (APRN) should discuss the potential for hemorrhage with patients at risk for developing a significant bleed and should reassure patients and families that if a significant bleed occurs, a plan of action will be promptly initiated.
- Spinal cord compression is a presenting symptom for 20% of cancer patients. It significantly affects quality of life, so the palliative APRN should maintain vigilance for its onset. With the exception of steroids, the palliative APRN must consider the patient's overall prognosis before initiating therapy.
- Seizures are a medical emergency. Brain metastases are the most common etiology of seizures in palliative care. In a patient experiencing seizures, death can occur from metabolic stress, rhabdomyolysis, lactic acidosis, aspiration pneumonitis, neurogenic pulmonary edema, and respiratory failure. Long-term empiric treatment with antiseizure medications is individualized based on the risk of seizure recurrence, the consequences of seizure recurrence, and potential interactions.
- Superior vena cava syndrome (SVCS) is a true medical emergency if the airway is obstructed. Lung cancer accounts for more than 70% of all cases annually. Early diagnosis and management can lead to a longer time between recurrences.

Hemorrhage

Although seen in people with advanced-stage diseases such as liver or lung disease, as well as in trauma, catastrophic bleeding is often due to a malignancy. Hemorrhage as a cause of death is relatively rare. Due to the lack of evidence, most management is based on case reports. Bleeding occurs in the form of nosebleeds, hemoptysis, hematemesis, rectal bleeding and melena, vaginal bleeding, direct arterial rupture, and fungating skin lesions/wounds. When bleeding occurs, the psychological effect on the patient, the family, and caregivers can be profound.

Identification of Patients at Risk

The pathophysiology of a bleed is related to the underlying cause or type of cancer a patient has. In patients with centrally located lung tumors, primarily bronchogenic carcinomas, hemoptysis or massive bleeding results from the creation of multiple collateral vessels, a buildup of vascular pressure, or direct invasion or treatment-related erosion of the bronchotracheal tissue.[1–3]

Patients with head and neck cancers are particularly susceptible, although specific statistics are unknown. Fungating tumors may directly invade the arteries in the neck.[4] Direct extension of tumor or damage to the wall of the artery by radiation therapy can weaken the wall, causing collapse. Radiation therapy is the primary cause of bleeding in this subset of cancer patients.[5] Surgery for this type of cancer carries risk as well, particularly in those undergoing radical neck dissection.

Causes of bleeding in patients with genitourinary malignancies are often the result of sloughing of the actual tumor mass, radiation-induced cystitis, and hemorrhagic cystitis from chemotherapy agents like cyclophosphamide.[6] Although it is rare, women with gynecologic cancers can have similar bleeding (bloody vaginal discharge) due to sloughing vaginal tissue or radiation therapy complications.[7] Bleeding from the gastrointestinal system can occur in people with primary cancers of the gastrointestinal system and are often complicated by disease involvement of the liver, which creates coagulopathies. Direct extension, seen in erosion of the wall of the esophagus, stomach, and small and large bowel, is always a possibility.

Treatment will depend on the underlying cause of the bleed, its extent, patient risk factors, and prognosis. Proactive planning about bleeding must occur. A bleeding event is frightening, so both patients and families need reassurance that it *can and will* be managed. This is particularly true if the patient has end-stage disease and desires care at home.[8]

Management

If bleeding occurs via the nose, rectum, or vagina, careful packing of the orifice can help. Hemostatic agents, such as alginates, are used with packing or compression dressings in vaginal packing to slow a bleed.[7] Agents like cocaine can be used with nasal packing.[7] Topical oxymetazoline (Afrin[R]) spray can be an inexpensive and effective method to stop many nosebleeds.[10] Bleeding surface wounds can be treated with hemostatic dressings, such as epinephrine or tranexamic acid syrup. However, limited data support the use of these agents in the control of severe surface wound bleeds.[1] Nonadherent dressings soaked in saline can provide a compression dressing and can, at times, slow or stop even arterial bleeding. A Wound Ostomy Certified Nurse (WOCN) can assist in making financially appropriate product choices since there are numerous supplies, many of them extremely costly.[1,11,12] Cauterizing or vasoconstricting agents are helpful for hemorrhagic cystitis, but these agents are contraindicated if the patient is also experiencing bladder spasm. A review of the literature reveals a lack of randomized clinical trials surrounding the management of hematuria.[6]

Endobronchial interventions, such as radiation therapy, can be tried if external-beam treatment is not effective. Endobronchial stenting has also been effective.[11,13] In addition to these active therapies, opioids control cough to minimize tracheal strain.[1,5] Patients who are bleeding from the skin, rectum, vagina, or bladder can benefit from a radiation oncology consult because external-beam radiation is highly effective at controlling bleeding from these sites.[5,6] For bleeding from the upper gastrointestinal tract, endoscopic interventions can stop or minimize bleeding and are considered to be the treatment of choice.[11,14] Laser coagulation, targeted cauterization of the bleeding lesion or vessels, and the injection of sclerosing agents directly into the site are effective in the management of gastrointestinal bleeds. Cystoscopic cautery is used in bladder cancer, usually after continuous bladder irrigation and lavage have proven ineffective. Bronchoscopy can be used in cases of refractory hemoptysis with topical applications of thrombin or fibrinogen, cold saline lavages, or laser phototherapy.[11]

Transcutaneous arterial embolization (TAE) may be employed to control bleeding in patients with metastatic hepatocellular bleeding. Embolization of the bilateral internal iliac arteries using permanent coils can be effective in patients with advanced urological cancer.[11,13]

Surgery is usually reserved for patients who have failed to respond to conservative attempts to control their bleeding and who can undergo a surgical procedure.

Phytonadione or vitamin K is important because it aids the liver in producing multiple clotting factors (II, VII, XI, X) if warfarin is found to be a causative therapy in a patient with bleeding or if malignancy has impaired the production of these factors.[11]

Vasopressin given either subcutaneously two or three times daily (not to exceed 600 mcg. per day) or via an intravenous continuous infusion at doses no greater than 50 mcg. per hour slows upper gastrointestinal bleeds as well as those caused by varices. Aminocaproic acid, a lysine analog, can be effective as medical management when bleeding occurs due to thrombocytopenias, hematological disorders, solid tumors, hepatic cirrhosis, complications of cardiac surgery, or any situation where fibrinolysis contributes to bleeding. Despite having medical management available, whenever possible, ligation of bleeding varices remains the most effective treatment.[1,11]

The use of platelet transfusions in a patient with any advanced malignancy depends on many factors, including the patient's prognosis and goals of care and the frequency of transfusions. Uncontrollable bleeding becomes most problematic when the platelet count falls below 20,000/mL[15] or, if a patient is afebrile and has no other coagulopathies, below 10,000/mL.[15]

Transfusions can have a positive effect on a patient's quality of life, but, as the need for infusions increases, frank discussions regarding the patient's goals of care are essential. The cessation of platelet transfusions is a difficult decision because, without them, life expectancy is limited.[16,17]

Anxiolytics, specifically fast-acting medications like midazolam and lorazepam, should be administered if a sudden bleed occurs. Midazolam is the drug of choice over lorazepam or diazepam because of its short half-life. It can be given intravenously or subcutaneously in the acute setting. In the home setting, however, lorazepam may be preferable due to the ease of administration via a butterfly needle device. A standard starting dose would be 2.5–5.0 mg every 10–15 minutes. Lorazepam can also be administered sublingually but will take longer to take effect. In the out-of-hospital setting, prefilled syringes of midazolam or lorazepam can be used and stored up to 13 days at room temperature. Opioids are suggested as second-line agents unless there is observable pain or increased work of breathing uncontrolled by midazolam.

Proactive Management of Hemorrhage

Depending on the site of bleeding, a terminal hemorrhage may cause death within moments and before any sedating medicine has taken effect. Proactive management should include the use of dark towels and sheets strategically placed near the patient. Family education should focus on the administration of opioids and anxiolytics if they observe any signs of distress in the patient. In the home setting, hospice services are an invaluable resource.

Spinal Cord Compression

Pathology

Spinal cord compression (SCC) is defined as a compression or invasion of the dural sac and the spinal cord by an extradural tumor mass or hematologically through Batson's venous plexus.[18] SCC most commonly occurs due to an extradural mass, which may be either osteolytic or osteoblastic. The neurological deficits that occur can be permanent due to direct compression of the cord or cauda equina, interruption of the vascular supply to the cord, or actual fracture of the vertebra. Less common etiologies are direct extension of the tumor through the intervertebral foramina or via leptomeningeal spread (most often seen in melanoma, lymphoma, and lung and breast cancer). The thoracic spine is affected in approximately 60% of all presentations. The lumbar spine accounts for 30% of all cases, followed by 10% in the cervical spine.[2,19] Spinal cord compression can occur in non-cancer conditions, such as osteoarthritis, rheumatoid arthritis, infection, any injury to the spine, and abnormal spinal alignment.[20–23]

Signs and Symptoms

Back pain, localized, mechanical, or radicular, is the most common presenting symptom, occurring in 83–95% of all cases of SCC and can precede other symptoms by 7 weeks.[19] It is especially important to consider SCC as a possibility in patients with thoracic pain. This is because this portion of the spine rarely is affected by pain-producing pathologies like osteoarthritis. Pain that occurs only with movement can be an important indicator of spinal instability, which might need rapid surgical intervention. Nonetheless, weakness with ambulation or the inability to walk combined with increased deep tendon reflexes offers the most significant predictor that the patient may be developing an SCC. While half of patients experience bladder dysfunction at the time of diagnosis,[19,24,25] this is considered to be a later sign of an SCC, as is bowel dysfunction.

A thorough physical exam includes gentle spine percussion to elicit pain. Changes in sensorium to heat and cold, vibration, light touch, coordination, gait, strength, and reflexes should be assessed. Sensory testing with neck flexion may reveal Lhermitte's sign (a shock-like sensation) that extends to the back, arm, and legs.[19,25] A saddle distribution of decreased sensorium below the level of the vertebrae can indicate cauda equina syndrome. Motor deficits are seen more in thoracic spread, while paresthesias and other sensory changes are seen in lumbar metastasis. Testing reflexes can indicate if nerve root compression could be affecting mobility and other motor movements.[19,24–26]

Diagnostics

Magnetic resonance imaging (MRI) of the entire spine is the gold standard of diagnosis. It should be ordered immediately when an SCC is suspected. Patients who have internal hardware may need a computed tomography (CT) scan with myelography for optimal spinal imaging. Myelography may also be more tolerable than MRI for a patient whose pain cannot be optimally controlled. Plain spinal radiographs are inappropriate.[25,27]

Management

A neurosurgery consult is imperative to determine what treatments are available. Other interventions include glucocorticosteroids, corticosteroids, radiation, and decompressive surgery. Spinal radiosurgery, percutaneous vertebroplasty, and kyphoplasty are common interventions. Both percutaneous vertebroplasty and spinal radiosurgery have been used in patients with SCC. Box 9.1 summarizes treatment recommendations for patients with an SCC.

Box 9.1 Summary Recommendations for Spinal Cord Compression

- Malignant spinal cord compression is a serious complication of cancer and should be treated as a medical emergency.
- Appropriate treatment depends on the patient's prognosis and the patient's and family's overall goals of care.
  - For patients with a life expectancy of days to a few months or those with complete paraplegia, appropriate treatments include pain management with opioids and consideration of steroids and single-fraction radiation therapy.
  - For patients with a life expectancy of months or longer who have a radiosensitive tumor, management should include immediate treatment with steroids followed by radiation therapy (either a short or longer course depending on the type of cancer).
  - For patients with a life expectancy of months or longer whose cancer is not radiosensitive, management should include immediate treatment with steroids followed by surgery. Radiation and/or chemotherapy may be considered after surgery if appropriate for the type of malignancy.

Supportive Therapies

Early entry into a physical medicine and rehabilitation (PM&R) setting suggests better outcomes.[28]

Seizures

Epilepsy is a disorder characterized by recurrent unprovoked seizures and categorized by its etiology as genetic, structural/metabolic, or unknown.[29] A seizure is considered a medical emergency.

Pathophysiology

Seizures are classified as focal, generalized, or psychogenic. Status epilepticus focal seizures consist of simple partial seizures without loss of consciousness or complex partial seizures with loss of consciousness. Generalized status epilepticus (tonic-clonic, absence/petit mal, myoclonic) seizures are always associated with loss of consciousness, and these have a greater incidence of associated mortality. Psychogenic status epilepticus is rare and characterized by bilateral rapid, jerky motor movements without loss of consciousness. When a seizure involves loss of consciousness, there will be a postictal state that may include somnolence, confusion, and/or headache; it may last several hours.[29]

Clinical Features

Factors influencing the risk of seizure recurrence include a history of long seizure duration and failure to respond to other medications.[30] Table 9.1 outlines predisposing factors for seizures.

Diagnosis

Status epilepticus of any type is determined by a neurological examination and involves repeated seizures lasting at least 5 minutes without a recovery

Table 9.1 Predisposing Factors for Seizures	
Factor	**Examples**
Structural	Brain tumor, metastasis, stroke, head trauma, subarachnoid hemorrhage
Degenerative	Cerebral palsy in young patients, Alzheimer's disease in older patients
Systemic	Cerebral anoxia/hypoxia or infections (such as encephalitis, meningitis, abscess), fever, sleep deprivation
Metabolic	Hepatic encephalopathy, uremia, electrolyte abnormalities, such as sodium, calcium, magnesium, phosphorus, or glucose abnormalities
Drug treatments	Use of seizure threshold-lowering drugs, such as antibiotics, antiarrhythmics, psychotropics, chemotherapy
Withdrawal	Rapid withdrawal from alcohol intoxication or antiseizure medications
From references 29, 31–33.	

Table 9.2 Suggested Postseizure Lab Testing

Test	Evaluation
CBC	Leukocytosis, thrombocytopenia, plethora
Blood chemistries	Ammonia, urea, sodium, calcium, magnesium, phosphorus, or glucose abnormalities
TSH	Low TSH indicates hyperthyroidism-associated seizures.
Urinalysis	Increased glucose, infection
C-reactive protein	Inflammatory marker; increased after tonic-clonic seizures
Coagulation studies	Increased risk of intracranial bleeding
Vitamin B_{12}, folate	Vitamin B_{12} deficiency, folate deficiency
Prolactin	Elevated levels seen after seizure
Blood cultures	Infectious cause
Blood gas	Hypoxia and metabolic imbalances
Toxicology	Overdose of tricyclic antidepressants, cocaine
Pregnancy test	Possible eclampsia

From reference 31.

period of greater than 30 minutes. Therefore, witnesses' accounts of activity prior to a seizure and description of seizure activity, including any incontinence or loss of consciousness, are crucial in determining the seizure type.

Management

Primary management when a seizure occurs includes the ABCs: patent airway, effective breathing, and adequate circulation. Table 9.2 summarizes suggested postseizure laboratory testing and the rationale. The American Academy of Neurology guidelines suggest prudent consideration of testing on an individual basis. When the seizure etiology is unknown, glucose and thiamine should be given together immediately to rule out treatable causes.[31]

Treatment of seizures should be initiated after 5 minutes of sustained seizure activity because they are unlikely to stop spontaneously (Table 9.3).

- First-line treatment of status epilepticus: 10 mg midazolam given intramuscularly or, more commonly, a 0.1 mg/kg bolus, usually 4 mg, of intravenous lorazepam.[31,37] Intravenous lorazepam has a rapid onset of 2–3 minutes and a long half-life of 4–12 hours.

- Second-line treatment of status epilepticus 10 mg diazepam given intravenously every 5 minutes until effective (maximum dose 40 mg) or a single 30 mg intrarectal gel, or midazolam 5–10 mg given intravenously or subcutaneously every 15 minutes up to a total of three doses.[38,39] Third-line treatment for status epilepticus is sedation (phenobarbital or propofol) inducing a chemical coma, with the goal to alleviate suffering while accepting the risk of respiratory failure.[31]

The decision to initiate long-term empiric treatment with antiseizure medication is individualized based on the risk of seizure recurrence, the consequences of seizure recurrence, and potential interactions.[34] After two or more unprovoked seizures on separate days, empiric monotherapy with

Table 9.3 Pharmacokinetic Characteristics and Other Administration Considerations of the Major Long-Term Antiseizure Drugs in Adults

Antiepileptic Drug	Usual Dosage (mg/day)	Therapeutic level (mg/L)	Common/Important Side Effects	Main Mechanism of Action	Peak Time (hours)	Half-Life (hours)	Protein Binding (%)	Metabolism and Excretion	Cost of Usual Starting Daily Dose for 1-Month Supply
Carbamazepine	400–2,400	4–12	Dizziness, drowsiness, nausea, leukopenia, aplastic anemia, hepatotoxicity, hyponatremia, Stevens–Johnson syndrome (SJS), toxic epidermal necrolysis (TEN)	Blocks voltage-dependent Na+ channels	4–8	5–26	75	Hepatic	$$
Clonazepam	0.5–4	0.02–0.08	Sedation, cognitive effects, drowsiness, respiratory depression	GABA receptor agonist	1–4	20–80	86	Hepatic	$
Felbamate	1,200–3,600	30–60	Hepatic failure, SJS, aplastic anemia, insomnia, weight loss, anorexia, nausea, headache	NMDA and Na+ channel conductance	2–6	13–30	25	Hepatic with renal excretion (40% as unchanged drug)	$$
Gabapentin	900–3,600	2–20	Weight gain, worsening of seizures, dizziness drowsiness, ataxia, peripheral edema	Blocks Ca+ channels, GABA receptor agonist	2–3	5–7	None	Renal excretion	$$
Lacosamide	200–400	10–20	Dizziness, headache, nausea, diplopia, blurred vision, cognitive dysfunction, skin reactions, ataxia	Slow inactivation of voltage-dependent Na+ channels	2–4	13	<15	Hepatic with renal excretion (40% as unchanged drug)	$$

Drug	200–600	1–15	Side effects	Mechanism	1–3	12–60	55	Metabolism	Cost
Lamotrigine	200–600	1–15	Rash, SJS, TEN, drug reactions with eosinophilia and systemic symptoms (DRESS), headache, blood dyscrasia, ataxia	Blocks voltage-dependent Na^+ channels	1–3	12–60	55	Hepatic with renal excretion (10% unchanged drug)	$$
Levetiracetam	1,000–3,000	3–30	Somnolence, asthenia, irritability, psychosis	Binding to synaptic vesicle protein 2	0.6–1.3	5–11	0 to <10%	Partially hydrolyzed in blood with 60% unchanged drug urinary excretion	$$
Oxcarbazepine	900–2,400	10–35	Somnolence, headache, diplopia, SJS, bone marrow suppression, hyponatremia	Blocks voltage-dependent Na^+ channels	4–6	8–10	38	Hydroxylation, glucuronidation with 95% urinary excretion	$$
Phenobarbital	30–180	15–40	Rash, sedation, dizziness, hepatotoxicity, impaired cognition, ataxia, mood change, SJS/TEN	GABA receptor agonist, glutamate antagonist, blocks voltage-dependent Na^+/Ca^+ channels	1–3	46–136	45–60	Hepatic	$
Phenytoin	150–600	10–20	Sedation, diplopia, hypotension with rapid IV administration, blood dyscrasia, hepatitis, SJS, gum hyperplasia, lupus-like reactions, hirsutism, acne, osteoporosis, cerebellar atrophy, peripheral neuropathy with chronic use	Blocks voltage-dependent Na^+ channels	4–12	24–72	85–95	Hepatic	$
Pregabalin	150–600	2–8	Somnolence, dizziness, ataxia	Binds to Ca^+ channels	1.5	6.3	None	Primarily eliminated unchanged in urine	$$

(continued)

Table 9.3 Continued

Antiepileptic Drug	Usual Dosage (mg/day)	Therapeutic level (mg/L)	Common/Important Side Effects	Main Mechanism of Action	Peak Time (hours)	Half-Life (hours)	Protein Binding (%)	Metabolism and Excretion	Cost of Usual Starting Daily Dose for 1-Month Supply
Topiramate	100–600	2–20	Impaired cognition, hepatotoxicity, weight loss, renal calculi, metabolic acidosis, anorexia	Blocks Na+ channels, GABA receptor agonist, blocks NMDA receptors	2–4	19–25	9–17	Minimal metabolism, 70% urinary excretion as unchanged drug	$$$
Valproic acid	500–2,500	50–100	Hepatotoxicity, pancytopenia, tremor, weight gain, hair loss, ovarian cystic syndrome, nausea, vomiting, anorexia	Increases availability of GABA (inhibitory neurotransmitter)	1–10	8–15	85–95	Hepatic	$
Vigabatrin	200–300	0.8–36	Visual field defects (33% permanent), fatigue, drowsiness, weight gain, edema, peripheral neuropathy	GABA transaminase inhibitor	1–2	6–8	None	Trivial metabolism, 80% urinary excretion as unchanged drug	$$$
Zonisamide	200–600	20–30	Somnolence, ataxia, dizziness, renal calculi, anorexia, headache, agitation, behavioral changes, word-finding difficulty	Blocks Na+ and Ca+ channels	2–6	60–70	40–50	Hepatic, 30% urinary excretion as unchanged drug	$$

Key: $, <$50; $$, $50–100; $$$, $100–500.
From references 34–36.

an antiseizure agent should be initiated to prevent recurrences. In seizures caused by a brain lesion, consider increasing or initiating steroids in addition to starting an anticonvulsant. Patients undergoing cerebral radiation should receive steroids (dexamethasone 4 mg to a maximum of 16 mg daily) to prevent seizures associated with cerebral edema.[40] If the patient is undergoing surgical resection of the brain tumor, then he or she may be weaned off antiseizure medications after surgery. If palliative chemotherapy is an option, preference should be given to antiseizure medications that do not induce cytochrome P450 activity; these include levetiracetam (Keppra), gabapentin (Neurontin), lamotrigine (Lamictal), and pregabalin (Lyrica).[40]

In the hospice setting, it is preferable to avoid enzyme-inducing medications or those that require following blood levels, such as phenytoin, phenobarbital, carbamazepine, oxcarbazepine, and topiramate.[34,40]

Superior Vena Cave Syndrome

Pathophysiology
The SVC is a thin-walled blood vessel. The brachiocephalic veins feed into the SVC, which terminates in the right atrium. An extrinsic chest mass generally to the right of midline (i.e., enlarged lymph nodes, lymphoma, thymoma, inflammatory process, or aortic aneurysm) or an internal thrombus compressing the SVC can easily cause obstruction of blood flow because the chest wall and surrounding organs leave little room for compensation. Increased venous pressure caused by the obstruction leads to increased flow through collateral blood vessels.

Clinical Features
SVCS classically presents as progressive swelling of the head and neck. Symptoms associated with increased venous pressure of the upper body usually develop over a period of 2 weeks and include edema of the face, neck, and arms. A blanching rash represents the excess development and dilation of compensatory subcutaneous vessels of the neck and anterior chest. SVCS can also manifest with cerebral edema, causing headaches, dizziness, and syncope or laryngopharynx-related compression, causing dysphagia, dyspnea, hoarseness, and cough.[41]

Diagnosis
Chest CT imaging with contrast is the most useful study to detect an impeding SVC compression, such as an aortic aneurysm or thrombosis, before symptoms present. MRI can be used when contrast medium is contraindicated. A tissue biopsy is recommended to diagnose malignancy.[42]

Management Strategies
To date, there are no evidence-based guidelines for the management of SVCS. Management of SVCS related to malignancy is guided by the severity of symptoms and anticipated response to the cancer. In all cases, the goal of treatment should be to alleviate bothersome symptoms of the obstruction. The American College of Chest Physicians and the National Comprehensive Cancer Network have made general recommendations supporting radiation

and stent placement for symptomatic SVC obstruction due to non-small cell lung cancer (NSCLC).

If thrombus is related to an indwelling catheter, anticoagulation is the primary treatment. Removal of the catheter and balloon dilation or stenting should be considered if fibrosis remains and is deemed clinically appropriate.[42,43] Placement of a stent has low risk and is optimal for symptom management of recurrent SVCS related to malignancy when the goal is to avoid the toxic effects of repeating chemotherapy or radiation.[44] Once a stent is placed, consideration should be given to anticoagulation and implications for management of SVCS recurrence, which occurs in an estimated 20–50% of patients. Researchers have used oral aspirin as antiplatelet preventive maintenance therapy after 3 to 4 days of complete heparinization after stent placement.[44]

References

1. Leigh A, Tucker R. What techniques can be used in the hospital or home setting to best manage uncontrollable bleeding. In: Goldstein N, Morrison R, eds. *Evidence-Based Practice of Palliative Medicine*. Philadelphia, PA: Elsevier Saunders; 2013:398–401.

2. Bobb BT. Urgent syndromes at end of life. In: Ferrell B, Coyle N, Paice J, eds. *Oxford Textbook of Palliative Nursing*. 4th ed. New York, NY: Oxford University Press; 2015:422–39.

3. Corey R, Hla KM. Major and massive hemoptysis: reassessment of conservative management. *Am J Med Sci*. 1987; 294: 301–9.

4. Powitsky R, Vasan N, Krempl G, et al. Carotid blowout in patients with head and neck cancer. *Ann Otol Rhinol Laryngol*. 2010; 119: 476–84.

5. Harris D, Noble S. Management of terminal hemorrhage in patients with advanced cancer: a systematic literature review. *J Pain Symptom Manage*. 2009; 38: 913–27.

6. Ghahestani SM, Shakhssalim N. Palliative treatment of intractable hematuria in context of advanced bladder cancer. *Urol J*. 2009; 6: 149–56.

7. Patsner B. Topical acetone for control of life-threatening vaginal hemorrhage from recurrent gynecologic cancer. *Eur J Gynaecol Oncol*. 1993; 14: 33–5.

8. McGrath P, Leahy M. Catastrophic bleeds during end-of life-care in haematology: controversies from Australian research. *Support Care Cancer*. 2009; 17(5): 527–37.

9. Hulme B, Wilcox S. *Guidelines on the management of bleeding for palliative care patients with cancer*. 2013; Yorkshire Palliative Medicine Clinical Guidelines Group, Yorkshire. http://www.palliativedrugs.com/download/090331_Summary_bleeding_guidelines.pdf. Accessed October 23, 2016.

10. Gilman C. *Focus on: treatment of epistaxis*. American College of Emergency Physicians. ACEP News. June 2009. Available at https://www.acep.org/Clinical---Practice-Management/Focus-On--Treatment-of-Epistaxis/ Accessed October 23, 2016.

11. Pereira J, Phan T. Management of bleeding in patients with advanced cancer. *The Oncologist*. 2004; 9: 561–70.

12. Alexander S. Malignant fungating wounds: managing pain, bleeding and psychological issues. *J Wound Care*. 2009; 18: 418–25.

13. Hague J, Tippett R. Endovascular techniques in palliative care. *Clin Oncol.* 2010; 22: 771–80.

14. D'Amico G, Pietrosi G, Tarantino I. Emergency sclerotherapy versus vasoactive drugs for variceal bleeding in cirrhosis: a Cochrane meta-analysis. *Gastroenterol.* 2003; 124: 1277–91.

15. Department of Health and Human Services -Tasmania Australia. *Care management guidelines: Emergencies in Palliative Care.* September, 2009 ed. Hobart, Tasmania: Tasmania: Department of Health and Human Services; 2009:1–12. Available at http://www.dhhs.tas.gov.au/palliativecare/health_professionals/symptom_management_guidelines. Accessed October 23, 2016.

16. Cartoni C, Delia M, Cupelli L, et al. Hemorrhagic complications in patients with advanced hematological malignancies followed at home: an Italian experience. *Leukemia & Lymphoma.* 2009; 50: 387–91.

17. Salacz ME, Lankiewicz MW, Weissman DE. Management of thrombocytopenia in bone marrow failure. *J Palliat Med.* 2007; 10: 236–244.

18. Nash R. What are the best pharmacological and surgical treatments for patients with spinal cord compression. In: Goldstein NM, ed. *Evidence-Based Practice of Palliative Medicine.* Philadelphia, PA: Elsevier; 2013:394–7.

19. Schiff D. *Clinical features and diagnosis of neoplastic epidural spinal cord compression, including cauda equina syndrome. UpToDate.* 2014; 1–15. http://www.uptodate.com/contents/clinical-features-and-diagnosis-of-neoplastic-epidural-spinal-cord-compression-including-cauda-equina-syndrome. Accessed October 23, 2016.

20. Williams K, Lin L, Cuccurullo SJ. Direct extension of a psoas muscle abscess leading to spinal cord compression. *Am J Phys Med Rehabil.* 2013; 92: 370.

21. Stoddard JE, Chiverton N. Thoracic facet joint synovitis causing thoracic spinal cord compression and myelopathy in a patient with rheumatoid arthritis. *Rheumatology.* 2011; 50: 2141–2.

22. Choi SH, Lee SH, Khang SK, Jeon SR. IgG4-related sclerosing pachymeningitis causing spinal cord compression. *Neurology.* 2010; 75: 1388–90.

23. Li MF, Chiu PC, Weng MJ, Lai PH. Atlantoaxial instability and cervical cord compression in Morquio syndrome. *Arch Neurol.* 2010; 67: 1530.

24. Loblaw DA, Perry J, Chambers A, Laperriere NJ. Systematic review of the diagnosis and management of malignant extradural spinal cord compression: the Cancer Care Ontario Practice Guidelines Initiative's Neuro-Oncology Disease Site Group. *J Clin Oncol.* 2005; 23(9): 2028–37.

25. Nash R. What are the signs and symptoms of spinal cord compression? In: Goldstein NM, ed. *Evidence-Based Practice of Palliative Medicine.* Philadelphia: Elsevier; 2013:390–3.

26. George R, Jeba J, Ramkumar G, Chacko AG, Leng M, Tharyan P. Interventions for the treatment of metastatic extradural spinal cord compression in adults. *Cochrane Database Syst Rev.* 2008(4): Cd006716.

27. Quraishi NA, Esler C. Metastatic spinal cord compression. *BMJ.* 2011; 342: d2402.

28. Fattal C, Fabbro M, Gelis A, Bauchet L. Metastatic paraplegia and vital prognosis: perspectives and limitations for rehabilitation care. Part 1. *Arch Phys Med Rehabil.* 2011; 92: 125–33.

29. Aminoff MJ, Kerchner GA. Nervous system disorders. In: McPhee SJ, Papadakis MA, eds. *2012 Current Medical Diagnosis and Treatment.* 51st ed. New York, NY: McGraw-Hill; 2012:942–9.

30. Alvarez V, Januel JM, Burnand B, Rossetti AO. Role of comorbidities in outcome prediction after status epilepticus. *Epilepsia*. 2012; 53: e89–92. doi: 10.1111/j.1528-1167.2012.03451.x

31. Benedict M, St. Louis EK. *Status epilepticus*. John Wiley & Sons. Available at http://www.essentialevidenceplus.com/content/eee/459. Accessed June 1, 2014.

32. Creutzfeldt CJ, Holloway RG, Walker M. Symptomatic and palliative care for stroke survivors. *J Gen Intern Med*. 2012; 27: 853–60. doi: 10.1007/s11606-011-1966-4

33. Canoui-Poitrine F, Bastuji-Garin S, Alonso E, et al. Risk and prognostic factors of status epilepticus in elderly: a case-control study. *Epilepsia*. 2011; 52: 1849–56. doi: 10.1111/j.1528-1167.2011.03168.x

34. Benit JP, Vecht CJ. Spectrum of side effects of anticonvulsants in patients with brain tumours. *Eur Assoc Neurooncol Mag*. 2012; 2: 15–24.

35. Lexi-Comp OnlineTM, *Lexicomp Drugs Online*.™ Hudson, OH: Lexi-Comp, Inc. http://www.wolterskluwercdi.com/lexicomp-online/ Accessed October 23, 2016.

36. Rogers SJ, Cavazos JE. Epilepsy. In: DiPiro JT, Talbert RL, Yee GC, Matzke GR, Wells BG, Posey LM, eds. *Pharmacotherapy: A Pathophysiologic Approach*. New York, NY: McGraw-Hill, 2014:855–82.

37. Silbergleit R, Durkalski B, Lowenstein D, et al. Intramuscular versus intravenous therapy for prehospital status epilepticus. *N Engl J Med*. 2012; 366: 591–600.

38. Brophy GM, Bell R, Claassen J, et al. Guidelines for the evaluation and management of status epilepticus. *Neurocrit Care*. Springer Science + Business Media LLC; 2012. doi: 10.1007/s12028-012-9695-2

39. Meirkord H, Boon P, Engelsen B, et al. European Federation of Neurological Societies (EFNS) guideline on the management of status epilepticus in adults. *Eur J Neurol*. 2010; 17: 348–55.

40. Tradounsky G. Seizures in palliative care. *Can Fam Physician*. 2013; 59: 951–5.

41. Ratnarathorn M, Craig E. Cutaneous findings leading to a diagnosis of superior vena cava syndrome: a case report and review of the literature. *Dermatology Online Journal*. 2011; 17: 4.

42. McCurdy MT, Shanholtz CB. Oncologic emergencies. *Critical Care Med*. 2012; 40: 2212–22.

43. Simoff MJ, Lally B, Slade MG, et al. Symptom management in patients with lung cancer: diagnosis and management of lung cancer, 3rd ed: American College of Chest Physicians evidence-based clinical practice guidelines. *Chest*. 2013; 143(5 Suppl): e455S–497S.

44. Lanciego C, Pangua C, Chacon JI, et al. Endovascular stenting as the first step in the overall management of malignant superior vena cava syndrome. *AJR Am J Roentgenol*. 2009; 193: 549–58.

Chapter 10

Discontinuation of Life-Sustaining Therapies

Kathy Plakovic

Key Points

- Withholding and withdrawing antibiotics, blood products, dialysis, and artificial nutrition are important topics that require shared decision-making.
- The benefits and burdens of treatment versus no treatment should be explained to the patient and family, along with the ethical framework that supports either decision.

Consensus Regarding Prognosis

The goal of withdrawing treatments is to allow the natural process of death to proceed instead of prolonging the dying process with treatments that may offer little benefit (and potentially high burdens) to the patient. It is important that there is consensus among healthcare providers regarding the prognosis before discussing it with patients and families. Obtaining consensus can be difficult because physicians are often overly optimistic in their prognosis.[1] Prognostic scoring systems, such as the Palliative Prognostic Score (PPS),[2] can assist clinicians in determining a prognosis for patients with diseases like cancer at the end of life.

Discussions should take place with patients and families regarding the prognosis with or without continued treatment. Patients with decision-making capacity can elect to forgo or withdraw life-sustaining treatment. For patients who lack capacity, their healthcare power of attorney or legal surrogate decision-maker can elect to withhold or stop treatment.

Antibiotics

Antibiotic use is common and is considered the standard of care for patients with an infection. Using antimicrobial medications at the end of life is a common practice.[3] As with other life-sustaining treatments, the decision to withhold or withdraw antibiotics requires informed decision-making based on the

Table 10.1 Likely Symptoms or Sequelae at End of Life	
Infection Site	**Associated Symptoms**
Urinary tract	Dysuria, fever, frequency, pain
Respiratory tract	Cough, dyspnea, fever, sputum production
Mouth/pharynx	Fever, mucosal inflammation/pain, odynophagia
Skin/subcutaneous	Fever, pain, skin rash/discoloration
Blood/bacteremia	Fever, disorientation, hypotension
Portions from reference 4. Reprinted with permission from Elsevier.	

goals of care for the individual patient. Table 10.1 offers the source of infections when considering continued antimicrobial use.

Blood Products

Transfusion of blood products, including red blood cells and platelets, is a life-sustaining treatment for patients with anemia and thrombocytopenia due to the disease process or treatment-related cytopenias. Often, many of these patients have hematologic malignancies and blood transfusions are a quality-of-life measure. Since their condition is difficult to predict, it is helpful to have a guideline to prognosis (Box 10.1). Many patients with advanced disease become transfusion-dependent due to bone marrow infiltration or chronic bleeding from tumor invasion. For these patients, continued transfusions are used not as a bridge to wellness but as a temporary measure.

Continuing transfusions in terminally ill patients can place a tremendous burden on the patient and family and usually requires frequent clinic visits for laboratory tests and transfusions, which can result in unplanned hospitalizations. Patients requiring frequent transfusions are at risk for fluid overload, transfusion reactions, and alloimmunization, making matched transfusions more difficult. Routine transfusions based on complete blood count results showing anemia or thrombocytopenia should be discouraged. Box 10.2 offers considerations for continued blood product use if a patient has end-stage disease.

Box 10.1 Prognostic Factors in Patients with Hematologic Malignancies

Eastern Cooperative Oncology Group (ECOG) status >2

Platelet count $<90 \times 10^{-9}$/L

LDH >248 U/L

Opioid use; World Health Organization (WHO) level 3

Albumin <30 g/L

Median survival with no or one risk factor, 440 days; two or three risk factors, 63 days; four or five risk factors, 10 days.

Adapted from reference 5. Reprinted with permission from Springer.

Box 10.2 Guidelines for Blood Product Use at End of Life

1. Exceedingly scarce resources, such as cross-matched and HLA-matched platelets, granulocytes, and rare units of blood should not be used in patients who have transitioned to palliative or comfort care. Routine blood products should be used sparingly, and requests should be reviewed by the transfusion medicine service.

2. Transfusions in medically futile situations should be avoided, if possible, and limited to the minimum number of red blood cell transfusions necessary to ameliorate symptoms of anemia. Platelets should also be limited to the minimum necessary to control bleeding or patient distress, such as upper airway bleeding. If the frequency of transfusions has an impact on the resources available for other patients (i.e., more than twice a week), the request should be reviewed by the transfusion medicine service.

3. If shortages of blood products arise, attempts should be made to defer transfusion in patients at the end of life, so the products can be used for other patients. Unusual requests, such as massive transfusion in a futile situation, are not indicated. If agreement cannot be attained in such situations, an ethics consult should be requested.

4. Transfusion in stable, terminally ill patients requires a careful analysis of the goals of care. Transfusions should not be discouraged in patients for whom an occasional transfusion is likely to alleviate primary symptoms, such as extreme fatigue. Large numbers of transfusions, however, should be reviewed by the transfusion medicine service.

Adapted from reference 6. Reprinted with permission from Wiley.

Dialysis

Use of the Renal Physicians Association/American Society of Nephrology *Guidelines for the Initiation and Withdrawal of Dialysis* can help guide discussions with patients and families regarding the appropriate time to start or stop treatment.[7] Prognosis can be difficult to predict for patients with end-stage renal disease (ESRD) once dialysis is initiated. Clearly, there is a survival benefit to initiating treatment versus withholding. However, discussing the short-term prognosis with patients and family members can aid in decision-making. Table 10.2 offers a mortality risk assessment for patients with ESRD.

It is important for patients and families to understand the prognosis with and without dialysis, so they can make informed decisions. Patients with ESRD who discontinued chronic dialysis had a mean survival of 7.8 days.[9] Patients with acute kidney injury (AKI) who withdraw from treatment have a much shorter life expectancy.[10] Patients and families can be counseled that death from uremia is usually peaceful because it induces coma. Symptoms like pain, myoclonus, dyspnea, or secretions can occur, and their management should be a priority.

| Table 10.2 Points Assigned to Each Risk Factor for Mortality in ESRD ||
Risk Factors	Points
Body mass index (kg/m²) <18.5	2
Diabetes	1
Congestive heart failure stage III or IV	2
Peripheral vascular disease stage III or IV	2
Dysrhythmia	1
Active malignancy	1
Severe behavioral disorder	2
Totally dependent for transfers	3
Initial context of dialysis unplanned	2

Adapted from reference 8. Reprinted with permission from Oxford University Press.

Nutrition

Families can have strong feelings about "feeding" patients and worry that without artificial nutrition the patient will "starve to death." Moreover, nutrition and eating and drinking may be considered a human right and part of reasonable care for patients. Nonetheless, total parenteral nutrition (TPN) has a limited role in advanced cancer patients. Bowel obstruction occurs in 25–50% of patients with advanced gynecologic cancers.[11] Venting gastrostomy tubes are commonly placed in patients with malignant bowel obstruction for symptomatic relief. There are conflicting data as to whether TPN after gastrostomy tube placement for bowel obstruction provides any survival benefit.

Anorexia is a natural part of the dying process. Patients generally lose their desire to eat as death nears. Often families will request enteral feeding via a nasogastric or percutaneous endoscopic gastrostomy (PEG) tube. The American Society of Parenteral and Enteral Nutrition (ASPEN) guidelines for nutritional support in cancer patients state that "the palliative use of nutrition support therapy in terminally ill cancer patients is rarely indicated."[32]

The burdens of continuing TPN include ongoing monitoring of laboratory values, electrolyte imbalances, and pancreatic and liver dysfunction,[13] as well as edema and worsening respiratory secretions. Patients also incur risks associated with ongoing central venous access, such as line infection leading to sepsis, thrombotic occlusion, and dislocation of the catheter.[14]

Conclusion

Life-sustaining treatments, such as antibiotics, blood products, dialysis, and artificial nutrition, can prolong the dying process in critically and terminally ill patients. These treatments may provide little benefit, and the burdens of these interventions can increase suffering. See Table 10.3 for consideration of withdrawal of these life-sustaining therapies.

Table 10.3 Sequelae of Withdrawal of Specific Life-Sustaining Therapies

Life-Sustaining Treatment	Likely Sequelae and/or Symptoms from Withdrawal
Antibiotics	Fever, delirium, cough, dyspnea, hypotension, somnolence
Blood products	Fatigue, weakness, shortness of breath
Dialysis	Pruritus, pain, myoclonus, dyspnea, secretions
Total parenteral nutrition	Hypotension, somnolence
Portions from reference 4. Reprinted with permission from Elsevier	

Families are often faced with decisions regarding withholding or withdrawing life-sustaining treatment as patients near the end of life. Recommendations regarding withholding or withdrawing treatments should be made based on medical knowledge and evidence-based practice.

References

1. Glare P, Sinclair C, Downing M, Stone P, Maltoni M, Vigano A. Predicting survival in patients with advanced disease. *Eur J Cancer.* 2008; 44(8): 1146–56.

2. Maltoni M, Scarpi E, Pittureri C, et al. Prospective comparison of prognostic scores in palliative care cancer populations. *Oncologist.* 2012; 17(3): 446–54.

3. Chun ED, Rodgers PE, Vitale CA, Collins CD, Malani PN. Antimicrobial use among patients receiving palliative care consultation. *Am J Hosp Palliat Care.* 2010; 27(4): 261–5.

4. Reinbolt RE, Shenk AM, White PH, Navari RM. Symptomatic treatment of infections in patients with advanced cancer receiving hospice care. *J Pain Symptom Manage.* 2005; 30(2): 175–82.

5. Kripp M, Willer A, Schmidt C, et al. Patients with malignant hematological disorders treated on a palliative care unit: prognostic impact of clinical factors. *Ann Hematol.* 2014; 93(2): 317–25.

6. Smith LB, Cooling L, Davenport R. How do I allocate blood products at the end of life? An ethical analysis with suggested guidelines. *Transfusion.* 2013; 53(4): 696–700.

7. Moss AH. Revised dialysis clinical practice guideline promotes more informed decision-making. *Clin J Am Soc Nephrol.* 2010; 5(12): 2380–3.

8. Couchoud C, Labeeuw M, Moranne O, et al. A clinical score to predict 6-month prognosis in elderly patients starting dialysis for end-stage renal disease. *Nephrol Dial Transplant.* 2009; 24(5): 1553–61.

9. O'Connor NR, Dougherty M, Harris PS, Casarett DJ. Survival after dialysis discontinuation and hospice enrollment for ESRD. *Clin J Am Soc Nephrol.* 2013; 8(12): 2117–22.

10. Dash T, Mailloux LU. *Withdrawal from and withholding of dialysis.* UpToDate, 2016. Available at http://www.uptodate.com/contents/withdrawal-from-and-withholding-of-dialysis?source=search_result&search=withdrawal+from+and+withholding+dialysis& selected Title=1%7E150. Accessed October 23, 2016.

11. Diver E, O'Connor O, Garrett L, et al. Modest benefit of total parenteral nutrition and chemotherapy after venting gastrostomy tube placement. *Gynecol Oncol*. 2013; 129(2): 332–5.

12. August DA, Huhmann MB. American Society of Parenteral and Enteral Nutrition clinical guidelines: nutrition support therapy during adult anticancer treatment and in hematopoietic cell transplantation. *J Parenter Enteral Nutr*. 2009; 33(5): 472–500.

13. Mirhosseini M, Fainsinger R. Fast Facts and Concepts #190,*Parenteral nutrition in advanced cancer patients*. 2015. Palliative Care Network of Wisconsin. Available at http://www.mypcnow.org/blank-cf128. Accessed October 23, 2016.

14. Dy SM. Enteral and parenteral nutrition in terminally ill cancer patients: a review of the literature. *Am J Hosp Palliat Care*. 2006; 23(5): 369–77.

Chapter 11

Withdrawal of Cardiology Technology

Patricia Maani Fogelman and Janine A. Gerringer

Key Points

- Heart failure advanced practice registered nurses (APRNs) are vital members of the management team for patients with heart failure. The heart failure and/or cardiac APRN is often the primary provider who maintains responsibility for managing the treatment of complex and advancing heart failure.
- The palliative APRN should anticipate and proactively manage symptoms associated with cardiac support discontinuation.
- Standardized protocols for withdrawal of life-sustaining respiratory therapies provide structured guidance, reduce variation in practice, and improve satisfaction of families and healthcare providers.

Discontinuation of Vasopressors

Vasopressors are medications delivered intravenously to support blood pressure during periods of hemodynamic instability in the acute care setting, most notably in the treatment of shock (Table 11.1).[1]

The general practice is to stop these medications when their desired effects are no longer elicited. The medications are withdrawn either at the same time or before or after ventilator support, without the need for medication weaning. Management of terminal heart failure symptoms (pain, dyspnea, nausea, anxiety) should be proactively addressed.

Discontinuation of Inotropes

Intravenous inotropic agents are used in acutely ill, hospitalized heart failure patients with a severely reduced ejection fraction. In the acute setting, inotropes are used to establish hemodynamic stability by increasing systemic perfusion and preserving end-organ function.

Inotropes may also be used as a long-term palliative treatment in patients whose advanced heart failure is refractory to other guideline-directed oral medications and who are not candidates for a ventricular assist device or a

Table 11.1 Vasopressors

Vasopressor Drug	Dose Range
Epinephrine	0.01–0.10 mcg/kg/min
Norepinephrine	0.01–3 mcg/kg/min
Phenylephrine	0.4–9.1 mcg/kg/min
Vasopressin	0.0–0.1 units/min
From reference 1.	

cardiac transplant. The goal of chronic inotrope therapy is symptom relief, and it is initiated based on hemodynamic evidence of clinical benefit and the patient's wishes. Goals of care and possible end-of-life scenarios should be discussed before starting continuous inotrope therapy.[2]

The most common inotropes used in the home setting are milrinone, dobutamine, and dopamine (Table 11.2). These inotropes can be administered intravenously through a small pump, which allows the patient to remain at home during treatment.[3]

Discontinuation of Ventricular Assist Devices

Mechanical circulatory support is becoming a widely accepted treatment for patients with advanced heart failure (stage D) with a reduced ejection fraction refractory to guideline-directed oral medications and cardiac device intervention. Ventricular assist devices (VADs) are designed to assist the patient's failing native ventricle by improving cardiac output.

VADs can serve patients in both the short term, when patients are acutely decompensated and hemodynamically unstable, and in the long term, when patients have chronic advanced heart failure. VADs can stabilize the patient so that decisions can be made regarding the plan of care, such as the need for surgical intervention (e.g., revascularization, correction of valve abnormalities, permanent pump placement, or, when appropriate, pump explant).[2]

Patients who are waiting for a cardiac transplant and need additional support until a donor heart becomes available can receive a left ventricular assist device (LVAD) as a bridge to transplant. If the patient's heart failure is severe and irreversible, and the patient is not a cardiac transplant candidate, he or she can receive an LVAD as destination therapy. Destination therapy with an LVAD has been proved to prolong survival and improve both quality of life and functional status in select patients with end-stage heart failure.[4]

Table 11.2 Inotropes

Inotropic Drug	Dose Range
Dobutamine	2.5–20 mcg/kg/min
Dopamine	5–20 mcg/kg/min
Milrinone	0.125–0.75 mcg/kg/min
From reference 2.	

Long-term LVADs are surgically implanted pumps that connect from the left ventricle to the ascending aorta to assist with systemic circulation. Blood exits the left ventricle through the inflow cannula, enters the pump, and is then directed through an outflow cannula to the aorta. An external driveline and power source are connected to the body to power the pump.[5]

When deactivating an LVAD, the patient's wishes need to be considered, wishes expressed directly through a living will or designated decision-maker. The medical team must agree on the lack of benefit of continuing device therapy in a patient with a minimal chance of meaningful recovery. If the interdisciplinary medical team cannot reach a consensus regarding device discontinuation, consultation with a hospital ethicist or ethics committee may be necessary.[6] See the companion volume to this book, *Advanced Practice Palliative Nursing* (2016), Chapter 48: Withdrawal of Cardiology Technology.

Petrucci and colleagues[7] provide a 10-point model for addressing ethical concerns in the treatment of VAD patients. Prior to deactivation of the LVAD, topics of discussion between the the patient and/or surrogate decision-maker should include current condition and prognosis, change in benefit of current therapy, how the device will be stopped, how symptoms will be treated, the patient's and/or surrogate decision-maker's readiness to proceed, and the anticipated outcome.[8] Different LVADs have different steps for deactivation. Healthcare professionals should first refer to any institutional protocols regarding VAD deactivation. In the absence of a formal institutional protocol, see Gafford and colleagues[9] for the key points for LVAD withdrawal and a peaceful death.

Deactivation can occur in the hospital or at home, depending on the patient's medical condition and wishes and whether the event is acute or chronic. In the hospital, the APRN can oversee the process and be available to support the patient and the staff. This includes writing orders for discontinuation of the device and administering medications for comfort. If deactivation is to occur at home, the APRN may teach the patient's family or hospice staff how to deactivate the device and administer medication for the patient's comfort to ensure a peaceful death.

Discontinuation of Pacemakers/Automatic Implantable Cardioverter-Defibrillators

Implantable pacemakers are commonly used to treat patients with symptomatic bradycardia and sinus node dysfunction. Current pacing systems have one or two leads that are positioned in the right atrium and right ventricle with a small computerized pulse generator that is placed under subcutaneous tissue in the shoulder area. The pacemaker can deliver an electrical pulse to the heart, leading to cardiac muscle contraction.[10]

Implantable cardioverter-defibrillators (ICDs) are devices that increase survival by terminating life-threatening arrhythmias. ICDs do not improve cardiac function or decrease symptom burden, but they decrease the risk of sudden cardiac death.[11] Cardiac resynchronization therapy (CRT), on the other hand, synchronizes segmental and global contraction of the left as well as the right ventricle in patients with systolic heart failure who have a left bundle-type wide

QRS complex and clinical symptoms of heart failure despite optimal medical therapy.[12] CRT can be combined with a pacemaker or ICD.[13]

CRT and ICD therapy may be available in the same device, but they offer very different options. CRT reduces the altered electrical activation of the left and right ventricles. The patient's goals of care should be assessed prior to implantation of a cardiovascular implantable electronic device (CIED; such as pacemaker or ICD). The healthcare provider is responsible for discussing both the risks and benefits of CIED therapy. Deactivation should be readdressed should any major changes occur in the patient's health status,[14] such as when prompted for a generator change, notification of device recall, diagnosis of another life-limiting illness, and when a decision is made for hospice care.[15]

Prior to device deactivation, the APRN should ensure that the patient understands his or her prognosis, any treatment options, and what will happen when the device is withdrawn and how deactivation of an automatic ICD may lead to death if a life-threatening arrhythmia occurs.[16]

Any provider or institution that implants CIEDs should have a protocol in place that clearly outlines the process for deactivating CIEDs when withdrawal of such care is appropriate. The final decision as to whether an ICD is burdensome should be made by the patient or a surrogate decision-maker.[17] Whenever possible, deactivation should be performed by healthcare professionals with electrophysiology experience, including physicians and device-trained nurses or technologists. In the absence of a device-trained specialist, deactivation can be performed by a healthcare professional such as a physician or a nurse under the guidance of an industry representative.[18] When a patient is at home with hospice or home healthcare, a pacemaker magnet can be used to deactivate an ICD generator if a programmer is unavailable.[9] Pacemakers may be withdrawn by changing the programming mode, or the rate may be lowered and the output adjusted so that the device is no longer functional. ICD deactivation can be performed by changing the programming or, for certain pulse generators, constant application of a magnet over the device. Placement of a magnet over a pulse generator of most ICDs will temporarily cease the anti-tachycardia therapies while not affecting the pacemaker function. To spare the patient from multiple painful shocks, a doughnut magnet and instructions for use should be provided to patients with a terminal diagnosis.[14] The patient should be reassured that deactivation of the ICD through reprogramming is not painful.[24] The defibrillator function of an ICD is separate from the pacing function. Pacing does not need to be disabled when the ICD is reprogrammed. Pacing may treat bradyarrhythmias and cardiac resynchronization at the end of life for symptomatic relief in patients without causing discomfort.[3]

Palliative Care and the Advanced Heart Failure Patient

Symptom Management

The predominant symptoms of distress for most dying patients, and especially those with cardiopulmonary organ failure, are pain, anxiety, and dyspnea.[19,20,21]

Morphine is the medication most commonly used to relieve pain and dyspnea in heart failure in the nonpalliative patient population presenting in florid distress.[22] The intravenous route is fastest for efficacy and relief in the acute inpatient setting, but for syndromes that become more chronic, oral regimens can be developed. Morphine is available in long-acting or short-acting tablet, liquid, and intravenous forms. See the companion volume to this book, *Advanced Practice Palliative Nursing* (2016), Chapter 23: Pain, and Chapter 24: Dyspnea, for further information.

Common symptoms to anticipate include chest pain, shortness of breath/dyspnea, air hunger, anxiety, nausea, and, later in the process, hallucinations. For patients with an LVAD, one of the most serious risk factors is a traumatic brain bleed leading to death. For these patients, control of neurotrauma-related symptoms is of utmost importance because they can often be most distressing to the family. Symptoms can include increased secretions, agitation, and myoclonic or seizure-like activity.

End-of-Life Medications Used in Cardiac Patients

In heart failure, the symptom prevalence is as follows: pain (78%), dyspnea (61%), depression (59%), insomnia (45%), anorexia (43%), anxiety (30%), constipation (37%), nausea/vomiting (32%), fatigue, difficulty ambulating, and edema.[21] Management includes the following therapies:

Lorazepam (Ativan)

Lorazepam is used to treat anxiety due to disease progression, uncontrolled dyspnea, or fear of dying. Cardiac patients become more dyspneic with disease progression, leading to increased levels of anxiety. They may have nausea from the effects of hypoperfusion and hypotension, for which lorazepam may also provide relief.[21] It can be given as an elixir, subcutaneously, intravenously, or as a continuous infusion for management of nausea, agitation, anxiety, myoclonus, or seizures.

Dosing varies based on the patient's history and needs. Begin at 0.5 mg intravenously or orally every 4 hours as needed and rapidly titrate up to an effective dose; doses may be needed every hour for some patients.[22,23]

Furosemide (Lasix)

Heart failure patients at the end of life often have fluid overload. Fluid status should be assessed prior to device removal. If fluid overload is noted, additional Lasix can be provided prior to withdrawal. Doses will vary because heart failure patients through the course of their illness tend to tolerate relatively high doses of diuretics. A urinary catheter may be used for comfort because frequent urination could create more distress than relief. To further reduce fluid overload, therapies that do not provide or contribute to comfort (e.g., intravenous fluids, continuous infusions) should be discontinued. Opioids, when given as an infusion, can be concentrated to limit unnecessary fluids.

Hyoscyamine (Levsin)

As their level of consciousness decreases, dying patients lose their ability to swallow and clear oral secretions resulting in gurgling or "rattling" noises. While there is no evidence that patients find this "death rattle" disturbing, the noises may be disturbing to family, visitors, or caregivers, who worry the patient is choking to death.

Hyoscyamine may be given orally or as an intravenous or subcutaneous injection for the management of oral secretions and is preferred over suctioning, which can cause further damage, swelling, edema, and secretions in the posterior airway and increase patient distress. Dosing generally begins at 0.125 mg.

Scopolamine (Transderm Scop)

An option for oral secretion management is scopolamine, which decreases secretions over a longer period of time. Because scopolamine takes 4 hours to hit peak effect, it is not useful for acute symptoms. The usual dose for scopolamine is a 1.5 mg patch replaced every 72 hours.[25]

Haloperidol (Haldol)

Haloperidol can be given as a liquid or as a subcutaneous or intravenous injection for management of agitation, restlessness, nausea, or terminal delirium. See the companion volume to this book, *Advanced Practice Palliative Nursing* (2016), Chapter 32: Delirium. Haloperidol is commonly used for sedation and is administered in a dose-escalation process similar to that used to treat pain: the starting dose is 0.5–2 mg given orally or intravenously every hour as needed.[22,23]

Conclusion

The management of heart failure begins with advance care planning. Early and ongoing discussions with patients and families are key. As heart failure worsens, the patient's needs will change, new symptoms will develop (or existing symptoms will intensify), and the goals of care may need to be revised. Keen assessment skills, partnership with palliative care, and close follow-up will ensure optimal symptom management. There is an art to balancing the needs of the patient and effective symptom management, and the assessment and management of symptoms go a long way to facilitate better quality of life.

References

1. Havel C, Arrich J, Losert H, Gamper G, Mullner M, Herkner H. Vasopressors for hypotensive shock. *Cochrane Database Syst Rev.* 2011; 5: 1–76.

2. Yancy CW, Jessup M, Bozkut B, et al. 2013 ACCF/AHA Guideline for the Management of Heart Failure: A Report of the American College of Cardiology Foundation/American Heart Association Task Force on Practice Guidelines. *Circulation.* 2013; 62(16): 1–6. Available at http://content.online-jacc.org/article.aspx?articleid=1695825. Accessed October 23, 2016.

3. Murthy S, Lipman HI. Management of end-stage heart failure. *Prim Care Clin Office Pract.* 2011; 38: 265–76.

4. Slaughter MS, Rogers JG, Milano CA, et al. Advanced heart failure treated with continuous flow left ventricular assist device. *N Engl J Med.* 2009; 361: 2241–51.

5. Slaughter MS, Pagani FD, Rogers JG, et al. Clinical management of continuous flow left ventricular assist devices in advanced heart failure. *J Heart Lung Transplant*. 2010; 29(1) Supplement: S1–S39.

6. Feldman D, Pamboukian SV, Teuteberg JJ, et al. The 2013 International Society of Heart and Lung Transplantation Guidelines for Mechanical Circulatory Support: executive summary. *J Heart Lung Transplant*. 2013; 32(2): 1–26.

7. Petrucci R, Benish LA, Carrow BL, et al. Ethical considerations for ventricular assist device support: a 10-point model. *ASAIO J*. 2011; 57: 268–73.

8. Allen LA. Stevenson LW, Grady KL, et al. Decision making in advanced heart failure: a scientific statement from the American Heart Association. *Circulation*. 2012; 125: 1928–52.

9. Wiegand DL, Kalowes PG. Withdrawal of cardiac medications and devices. *AACN Adv Crit Care*. 2007; 18(4): 415.

10. Kusumoto FM, Goldschlager N. Device therapy for cardiac arrhythmias. *JAMA*. 2002; 287(14): 1848–52.

11. Bardy GH, Lee KL, Mark DB, Poole JE, Boineau R, Domanski M. Amiodarone or an implantable cardioverter-defibrillator for congestive heart failure. *N Engl J Med*. 2005; 352(3): 225–37.

12. Jarcho JA. Biventricular pacing. *N Engl J Med*. 2006; 355: 288–94.

13. Kramer DB, Reynolds MR, Mitchell SL. Resynchronization: considering device-based cardiac therapy in older adults. *J Am Geriatr Soc*. 2013; 61: 615–21.

14. Lampert R, Hayes DL, Annas GJ, et al. HRS Expert Consensus Statement on the Management of Cardiovascular Implantable Electronic Devices (CIEDs) in patients nearing end of life or requesting withdrawal of therapy. *Heart Rhythm*. 2010; 7(7): 1008–26.

15. Morganweck CJ. Ethical considerations for discontinuing pacemakers and automatic implantable cardiac defibrillators at end-of-life. *Curr Opin Anesthesiol*. 2013; 26: 171–5.

16. Swetz KM, Freeman MR, Abou-Ezzeddine OF, et al. Palliative medicine consultation for preparedness planning in patients receiving left ventricular assist devices as destination therapy. *Mayo Clin Proc*. 2011; 86(6): 493–500.

17. Wiegand DL, Kalowes PG. Withdrawal of cardiac medications and devices. *AACN Adv Crit Care*. 2007; 18(4): 415–25.

18. Lindsay BD, Estes MNA 3rd, Maloney JD, Reynolds DW. Heart Rhythm Society Policy Statement Update: recommendations on the role of Industry Employed Allied Professionals (IEAPs). *Heart Rhythm*. 2008; 5(11): e8–10.

19. Mularski RA, Reinke LF, Carrieri-Kohlman V, et al., on behalf of the ATS Ad Hoc Committee on Palliative Management of Dyspnea Crisis. An Official American Thoracic Society Workshop Report: assessment and palliative management of dyspnea crisis. *Ann Am Thorac Soc*. 2013; 10(5): S98–106.

20. Whellan DJ, Goodlin SJ, Dickinson MG, et al.; Quality of Care Committee, Heart Failure Society of America. End-of-life care in patients with heart failure. *J Card Fail*. 2014; 20(2): 121–34. doi: 10.1016/j.cardfail.2013.12.003.

21. Reisfield GM, Wilson GR. Fast Facts and Concepts #144.*Palliative care issues in heart failure*. 2015. Palliative Care Network of Wisconsin. Available at http://www.mypcnow.org/blank-fmfev. Accessed October 23, 2016.

22. Chou R, Fanciullo GJ, Fine PG, et al; American Pain Society-American Academy of Pain Medicine Opioids Guidelines Panel. Clinical guidelines for the use of chronic opioid therapy in chronic noncancer pain. *J Pain*. 2009; 10(2): 113–30.

23. American Pain Society. Herdon C, Arnstein P, Darnall B, Hartrick C, Hecht K, Lyons M, Maleki J, Manworren R, Miaskowski C, Sehgal N, eds. *Principles of Analgesic Use in the Treatment of Acute Pain and Cancer Pain*, 7th ed. Chicago, IL: American Pain Society; 2016.

24. Goldstein N, Carlson M, Livote E, Kutner JS. Brief Communication: management of implantable cardioverter-defibrillators in hospice: a nationwide survey. *Ann Intern Med.* 2010; 152: 296–9.

25. Hirsch CA, Marriott JF, Faull CM. Influences on the decision to prescribe or administer anticholinergic drugs to treat death rattle: a focus group study. *Palliat Med.* 2013; 27(8): 732–8. doi: 10.1177/0269216312464407.

Chapter 12

Withdrawal of Respiratory Technology

Beth Wagner

Key Points

- Respiratory failure and pulmonary advanced practice registered nurses (APRNs) are vital members of the management team for patients with heart failure and pulmonary failure.
- The palliative APRN should anticipate and proactively manage symptoms associated with discontinuation of respiratory support.
- Standardized protocols for withdrawal of life-sustaining respiratory therapies provide structured guidance, reduce variation in practice, and improve satisfaction of families and healthcare providers.

Guidelines for Withdrawal of Respiratory Support

The majority of deaths in the intensive care unit (ICU) occur after decision to limit or withdraw life-sustaining therapies.[1] Death often occurs rapidly following the removal of respiratory life support, which places a great burden of decision on families and care providers.[2] Removing life-sustaining therapy involves complex decisions filled with a myriad of emotions for all involved.

Consensus guidelines have emerged to promote quality and improve end-of-life care for critical care patients.[3,4] Box 12.1 lists essential steps to include in clinical pathways, multidisciplinary care plans, or protocols to provide guidance for the care of patients when respiratory life support is withdrawn.

Oxygen

The choice of an oxygen delivery system depends on numerous factors, including disease state, clinical status, amount of oxygen required, and patient comfort and acceptance. The goals of oxygen therapy are to attain adequate resting oxygen levels to prevent damage to the tissue from hypoxia, to minimize the risk of oxygen-induced injury, and to provide symptom relief. In general, an oxygen saturation (SpO_2) of more than 90% or a partial pressure of

> ### Box 12.1 Steps for Terminal Weaning from Mechanical Ventilation
>
> - Ensure patient's comfort prior to initiating.
> - Reduce fraction of inspired oxygen (FiO_2) to 21% or room air and remove positive end-expiratory pressure (PEEP). Observe for signs of respiratory distress. Adjust opioids and benzodiazepines.
> - Reduce intermittent mandatory ventilation (IMV) rate and/or PS to 4–6 over 5–20 minutes. Observe for signs of respiratory distress. Adjust medication.
> - Deflate endoctracheal tube (ETT) cuff if present.
> - Silence alarm; turn off ventilator.
> - Disconnect tubing from the tracheostomy or remove the ETT while covering with a clean towel that will collect the secretions as well as hide the ETT. If not removing the ETT, disconnect connection to ventilator and apply T-piece with humidified air.
> - If oropharyngeal secretions are present, suction gently. Avoid deep suction.
> - Oxygen is not necessary.
> - Move ventilator out of room.
> - Encourage family to touch and hold patient. Some may want to lie in bed beside the patient.
>
> From references 2, 5, and 6.

oxygen in arterial blood (PaO_2) of more than 60 mm Hg is adequate to meet metabolic demands. Specific goals are individualized for specific disease states or severity of illness, such as chronic obstructive pulmonary disease (COPD) and acute respiratory distress syndrome (ARDS).

A nasal cannula is the most commonly used method to provide supplemental oxygen in the hospital or ambulatory setting.[7] Both low- and high-flow oxygen rates can be delivered by nasal cannula. The initial nasal cannula design provided only low-flow oxygen, with flow rates up to 6 L per minute. In this system, 100% oxygen is directed through a bubbler humidifier at a rate of approximately 1–6 L per minute. The oxygen mixes with inspired air, resulting in delivery of an oxygen concentration of approximately 25–40% depending on patient's respiratory rate, tidal volume, and use of mouth breathing.[8] Oxygen is used to alleviate dyspnea in people with COPD with severe hypoxia, but there is sparse evidence that oxygen relieves breathlessness in mild hypoxemic or non-hypoxemic conditions.[9]

There is no support for the initiation or continuation of oxygen therapy when the patient is non-hypoxemic or comfortable and near death.[10] The use of a fan directed toward the patient's face or cognitive-behavioral therapy can diminish breathlessness.[9,11]

The high-flow nasal cannula oxygen (HFNCOx) system involves delivery of heated and humidified oxygen via specialized oxygen blenders that are capable of flow rates of 8 L per minute in infants and up to 60 L per minute in children and adults. In addition, HFNCOx generates a low level of positive airway pressure with greater ease of use and patient comfort compared to therapies with tight face masks, such as bilevel positive airway pressure (BiPAP).[12] HFNCOx maintains an elevated FiO_2 by using high flow rates to increase arterial oxygenation and promote nasopharyngeal washout of entrapped room air, resulting in decreased upper airway resistance and work of breathing.[13] The components of a HFNCOx system include a patient interface, a gas delivery device to control flow and FiO_2, and a humidifier. Unlike non-rebreather systems, high-flow oxygen therapy systems use a nasal cannula, allowing patients to talk and eat while receiving high-flow oxygen; this contributes to their improved tolerability and acceptance.

There is a trend toward using HFNCOx as an alternative to noninvasive positive-pressure ventilation for patients with a "do not intubate" status who are receiving comfort-only care.[12] The clinical indications or guidelines for use, however, are not yet clearly established.[13]

Because oxygen levels naturally will decrease in all imminently dying patients, oxygen provides little to no palliative benefit. The removal of the oxygen may promote interaction between the patient and loved ones because the patient's face is no longer encumbered by tubes or masks. If patients are awake, they may be able to express their preference for removal of the oxygen. That discussion should include assurance to the patient and family that the symptom of breathlessness will be controlled in either approach. Low-flow oxygen can be provided in any setting. HFNCOx requires specialized air compression systems to generate the high flow rates, and these are primarily available only in acute care settings and generally not in the home or hospice.

A major challenge arises for patients in the acute care setting who are receiving HFNCOx and who are stable but cannot progress with weaning. With increasing reports of positive outcomes with the use of HFNCOx, more patients are placed on HFNCOx but then do not improve. Because of its limited availability outside the acute care setting, these patients are often faced with the decision to discontinue HFNCOx therapy. Therefore, when contemplating the application of HFNCOx, it should be considered to be like any other form of life support, and a discussion of the goals of care and benefit versus burden should precede its use. New technology is emerging for the administration of HFNCOx in the home or hospice. However, due to the very specialized equipment and high costs, it is unlikely that in the near future it will be routinely available in hospice care. For patients who want to die at home, the benefits and burdens of HFNCOx therapy need to be addressed.

There are no specific evidence-based guidelines for discontinuation of either high- or low-flow oxygen. Patients requiring HFNCOx to maintain adequate oxygenation saturation levels will likely experience dyspnea upon withdrawal.

Mechanical Ventilation

Mechanical ventilation involves the support of breathing by means of an external machine in patients with respiratory failure. It can be provided either by an invasive technique, such as endotracheal intubation, or a noninvasive technique, such as noninvasive positive-pressure ventilation (NPPV) through a mask applied to the mouth or nose. The indications for mechanical ventilation include the inability to sustain adequate oxygenation, the need for the elimination of carbon dioxide, or maintenance and protection of the airway. Any decision to initiate mechanical ventilation should be preceded by a discussion with the patient and/or family that reviews the goals of care, the benefits and burdens of the intervention, and alternative treatment options.

Invasive Mechanical Ventilation

Invasive mechanical ventilation provides gas exchange in the lungs with an artificial airway that is established via an endotracheal or tracheostomy tube. A large-bore flexible tube is used as the interface between the ETT or the tracheostomy tube and the ventilator. Orotracheal intubation is the most common method of inserting an ETT, but nasotracheal intubation is also possible to maintain the patency of the upper airway. Endotracheal intubation is considered a relatively temporary procedure because long-term use increases the risk of complications related to cuff pressures or erosion caused by the tube. Guidelines suggest that patients should not be ventilated via an ETT for longer than 3 weeks. Through an incision into the trachea, a tracheostomy tube is surgically placed to provide long-term airway access.

Detailed planning for withdrawal of invasive mechanical ventilation at the end of life ensures the patient's comfort during the process. Steps for a gradual wean based on principles and recommendations from the literature are outlined in Table 49.1.[2,5,6] There are two methods of ventilator withdrawal: (1) rapid or immediate cessation of mechanical ventilation, sometimes referred to as terminal extubation, and (2) terminal weaning, which is the gradual, stepwise withdrawal of ventilation, with assessment and interventions for discomfort before moving to the next step. No evidence supports one method over another nor the removal of the ETT and extubation. Patients experiencing bleeding in the upper respiratory tract, stridor, excessive secretions, and occlusion secondary to external compression by a tumor or a swollen tongue are at greater risk for airway compromise if the tube is removed. Leaving the tube in place may be a source of discomfort to patients as well as a physical barrier that prevents face washing, mouth care, and touching or kissing the face.

NPPV

NPPV refers to assisted ventilation by the application of BiPAP delivered through an externally placed mask, mouthpiece, or helmet apparatus. The oronasal mask is generally preferred over a nasal mask or nasal prongs during the initiation of NPPV. The full-face mask may be an option for patients who experience discomfort, such as excessive device pressure, or fail to achieve adequate improvement in gas exchange. The use of NPPV has gained increasing acceptance as a first-line therapy for patients with acute respiratory failure to temporize pulmonary status while treating the patient to avoid endotracheal intubation. It is less invasive, often requires less sedation, and is associated with lower rates of ventilator-associated pneumonia than endotracheal intubation.

The use of NPPV can reduce the rate of endotracheal intubation by providing additional time to assess and correct a reversible process.

Conditions known to respond to NPPV include exacerbations of COPD, respiratory failure in immunocompromised patients and cardiogenic pulmonary edema, and amyotrophic lateral sclerosis (ALS).[14] It can be an effective stabilizing measure for a patient who prefers to remain more alert or to delay death until family or loved ones can arrive at the bedside.[15]

Relative contraindications for the use of NPPV include facial trauma or anatomy limiting placement of the mask; inability of the patient to cooperate, protect the airway, or clear secretions; high aspiration risk; severely impaired consciousness; recent esophageal anastomosis; and upper airway obstruction.[16] Factors that may reduce the tolerance or acceptance of therapy include discomfort from a tight-fitting mask or high-pressure air flow, facial skin breakdown, claustrophobia, anxiety, aspiration, dryness of mucous membranes, loud noise of the machine, and interference with communication and family intimacy. Small doses of a benzodiazepine can alleviate anxiety.

At the time of withdrawal of NPPV, patients may experience significant respiratory distress.[17,18] Removal of NPPV requires many of the same considerations as ETT removal. Prior to weaning NPPV, the initiation of opioids and benzodiazepines is appropriate to decrease dyspnea and anxiety.

There are no evidence-based protocols for weaning NPPV at the end of life. Common practice employs incremental reduction of the inspiratory positive airway pressure (iPap) by 2 cm H_2O, in conjunction with gradual reduction in FiO_2. The backup rate setting, which triggers an automatic cycle on some machines if a patient does not spontaneously take a breath, can be turned off in dying patients. Once the iPap is approximately 6 cm H_2O or less above expiratory positive pressure and the patient is comfortable, NPPV can be removed. There is no evidence to support automatic placement of nasal cannula oxygen when NPPV is removed in an end-of-life scenario.

Extracorporeal Life Support

Extracorporeal life support (ECLS), also known as extracorporal membrane oxygenation (ECMO), provides continuous cardiopulmonary support for a temporary period, typically days to weeks, as supportive management of severe respiratory and/or cardiac failure. This technique uses a modified heart-lung bypass machine that pumps and oxygenates a patient's blood, thus allowing the heart and lungs to rest. The purpose of ECLS is to facilitate recovery of the lungs and heart by minimizing ventilator-induced lung injury while allowing additional time to diagnose and treat the underlying disease.

ECLS accomplishes bypass of the normal heart-lung circulation through a device (called "the circuit") that transports the blood outside the patient's body through an artificial lung. The artificial lung contains two compartments separated by a gas-permeable membrane, with the blood on one side and the ventilating gas on the other, where carbon dioxide is extracted and the blood is oxygenated. It is then warmed and returned to the heart. The two most common configurations of ECLS are veno-arterial (V-A) and veno-venous

(V-V). The V-A configuration provides both cardiac and respiratory support. Blood is withdrawn from venous circulation and returns to arterial circulation through either peripheral or central cannulation. Femoral venous and femoral arterial cannulation are preferred in adult patients.[19] The V-V configuration drains blood from the venous circulation; it is returned to the venous circulation close to the right atrium through peripheral cannulation, typically using the right internal jugular and/or femoral veins in adults. The V-V configuration provides respiratory support only, with no hemodynamic support, and therefore is used when the heart is functioning well and only the lungs require support. If only respiratory support is needed, this method is preferred because it reduces the risk of complications associated with arterial cannulation, such as limb ischemia and thrombotic or air emboli.

ECLS has been instituted for cardiac support in patients who cannot be removed from cardiopulmonary bypass following cardiac surgery, post heart transplant with primary graft failure, and severe cardiac failure due to other causes, such as sepsis, decompensated cardiomyopathy, myocarditis, and drug overdose. In addition, ECLS is used to provide support for patients as a bridge to either placement of a ventricular assist device or cardiac transplantation. Common indications for patients requiring pulmonary support include respiratory failure due to pneumonia, ARDS, trauma, or primary graft failure following lung transplant. ECLS for influenza has been performed in neonatal and pediatric populations, with an overall survival rate to discharge of 50%.[19] In patients with the V-V configuration, the trial off the system is relatively simple. Venous and arterial cannulas placed by percutaneous access can be removed directly and bleeding controlled by application of direct pressure. Cannulas placed by direct cutdown are removed by direct cutdown, with ligation of the vessel if needed. Femoral artery cannulation by cutdown requires vascular repair at the time of cannula removal.

Guidelines from the Extracorporeal Life Support Organization (ELSO) list criteria (Box 12.2) to consider in the determination of futility and discontinuation of ECLS.[20]

Drug sequestration by the ECLS circuit has been observed with several medications, including some commonly used for end-of-life symptom management, such as opioids (morphine, fentanyl), benzodiazepines (midazolam,

Box 12.2 Criteria for Determination of Futility and Discontinuation of ECLS (ELSO Guidelines)

Severe brain damage

No cardiac function after 3 days in a patient who is not a ventricular assist device or transplant candidate

No lung function after 14–50 days in a patient who is not a transplant candidate

Fixed pulmonary hypertension after several weeks

Uncontrolled bleeding

Other irreversible organ failure

Note: The definition of irreversible heart, lung, or brain damage will vary by institution.

diazepam, lorazepam), and propofol. It can later result in a prolonged release of the drug from the circuit after the drug is stopped. This presents significant challenges for effective dosing of the analgesics and sedatives necessary to provide comfort in patients undergoing ECLS. Lipophilic drugs, such as fentanyl, and highly protein-bound drugs are significantly sequestered in the circuit, leading to suboptimal drug concentrations in the body.[21] For this reason, it appears that morphine, a hydrophilic drug, may be superior to fentanyl in patients on ECLS.[21] Because of numerous variables affecting the sequestration of drugs and rapid advances in the technology, simply increasing the dose administered is not effective and may result in toxic levels.

Prostacyclin Therapy

Prostacyclin therapy is commonly used in the treatment of pulmonary arterial hypertension (PAH) as a palliative measure to extend life and control symptoms. PAH is a progressive, terminal illness characterized by dysfunction of the pulmonary arteries. Vasoconstriction and vascular hypertrophy within the pulmonary artery lead to restriction of blood flow, which increases peripheral vascular resistance and eventually right-sided heart failure. Exertional dyspnea with exercise intolerance is the most common and debilitating symptom of PAH. The goal of therapy for PAH is to slow disease progression and control exertional dyspnea by lowering pulmonary arterial pressure and pulmonary vascular resistance.

Prostacyclin is a naturally occurring prostaglandin that inhibits the aggregation of platelets and is a potent vasodilator used in the treatment of advanced PAH. Currently, three prostacyclin analogues are used in the treatment of PAH: treprostinil (Remodulin), iloprost (Ventavis), and epoprostenol (Flolan, Veletri). Treprostinil is available in intravenous, subcutaneous, or inhaled formulations. Iloprost is administered via inhalation. Epoprostenol has a very short half-life of approximately 6 minutes, so it can be administered only via continuous intravenous infusion. Prostacyclin therapy can be administered in the home, but the complexity of epoprostenol infusion can be arduous for patients and their caregivers.

Prostacyclin therapy presents unique challenges with respect to end-of-life issues. It is a life-sustaining therapy that may be needed for prolonged periods of time. Abrupt withdrawal, large reductions in dosage, or interruptions in drug delivery can lead to sudden rebound pulmonary hypertension and severe respiratory distress. Most patients with PAH die in the ICU.[22] De-escalation of intravenous prostacyclin should occur in a setting with close medical supervision, knowledgeable staff, and sufficient amounts of readily available medications to allow for rapid adjustments and administration to ensure symptom management and comfort.

Recommendations suggest the reduction of the prostacyclin in 10–25% increments.[22,23] The medication's half-life affects the rate of taper. Epoprostenol, with a half-life of approximately 6 minutes, can be tapered every 25–30 minutes. Treprostinil infusion has a longer half-life of approximately 4 hours, but significant increases in pulmonary pressures were noted within 1 hour of treprostinil discontinuation.[23] A reasonable approach is to reduce the treprostinil infusion every 4–6 hours. The patient is closely monitored for symptoms with each dose reduction.

Symptom Control During Withdrawal of Respiratory Life-Sustaining Therapies

When the decision has been made to discontinue respiratory support, the initial critical step is to establish the plan for adequate symptom control prior to the extubation. Common symptoms related to withdrawal of respiratory life support include dyspnea, anxiety, accumulation of pulmonary secretions, and dry mouth. Management of symptoms not only is essential for comfort, but also to relieve the family's perceptions and level of distress.[24,25]

The Respiratory Distress Observation Scale (RDOS) is a validated tool often used in the ICU to measure and show trends in respiratory distress and response to treatment in adults (Box 12.3).[26]

Neuromuscular blocking agents interfere with the ability to assess the patient's comfort because they mask objective signs of discomfort, such as grimacing and tachypnea; therefore, such agents may contribute to patient suffering. These agents should be discontinued prior to life support withdrawal, allowing sufficient time for clearance of the drug, which may be influenced by liver and renal function.

Opioids and benzodiazepines are supported by the most evidence as a means to relieve dyspnea at the end of life. See the companion volume to this book, *Advanced Practice Palliative Nursing* (2016), Chapter 24: Dyspnea. There is disagreement on the use of opioids in the severely neurologically impaired patient. It is unclear if the absence of distress indicators is a result of the patient's inability to perceive discomfort or the inability to manifest the signs. This raises uncertainty for clinicians, resulting in variability in practice. Some suggest that the administration of sedatives and opioids is still guided by the presence of patient behaviors.[27] Others recommend administration

---

Box 12.3 Objective Correlates of Discomfort

Grimacing

Tachypnea

Tachycardia

Restlessness or agitation

Fearful facial expression

Accessory muscle use (rise and fall of clavicle)

Paradoxical breathing

Nasal flaring

Moaning

Grunting at end-expiration

From reference 26.

Table 12.1 Recommended Initial Parenteral Bolus Dose of Opioid in Opioid-Naïve Patients	
Opioid	**Initial Bolus Dose**
Morphine	2–10 mg
Hydromorphone	0.2–0.6 mg
Fentanyl	50–100 mcg

of the average doses cited in studies, with adjustments in those doses only if behavioral signs of clinical distress occur during the withdrawal process.

Patients should be made comfortable prior to weaning or removing the respiratory support therapy. In some patients, symptoms can be controlled with intermittent doses of an opioid. A continuous opioid infusion should be used for patients who are already experiencing dyspnea, or if it is anticipated that the patient's dyspnea will worsen. For patients who are naïve to opioids, opioid initiation can begin with the recommended bolus doses listed in Table 12.1. If initiating an infusion, guidelines generally suggest beginning with a bolus dose and initiating the infusion at a rate 50–100% of the bolus dose. For example, if the bolus dose is morphine 10 mg given intravenously, the infusion would begin at 5 mg per hour.

If the patient is already receiving opioids, a bolus of two times the current hourly rate should be administered, and then the continuous infusion rate should be increased by 25%. Increases in doses should be preceded by a bolus so that steady-state levels are achieved rapidly. Increasing the infusion rate alone can significantly prolong the time to achieve patient comfort. The common bolus dose of morphine is 5–10 mg given intravenously (or another opioid at equianalgesic doses) or 10% of the patient's daily opioid dose every 10 minutes, as needed, to keep the respiratory rate under 28 breaths/minute with no evidence of other behavioral correlates of distress. The continuous infusion rate should be increased by 25% if the patient requires more than two bolus doses within an hour. Implementation of a standardized order form, with guidelines for titration of medications, improved caregiver satisfaction and increased the use of opioids and benzodiazepines, without significant decrease in the time from withdrawal of mechanical ventilation to death.[5]

Additional Symptoms

Stridor is a harsh, high-pitched breath sound resulting from a narrowed or obstructed airway that can occur in patients with respiratory failure. The underlying cause can be extrinsic compression by a tumor, edema of the head and neck, or central airway obstruction. Stridor can be disconcerting to the care providers and family because they may perceive that the patient is choking and suffering. Suggestions for prevention or palliation of stridor include racemic epinephrine or corticosteroids.[28,29] In adults, multiple doses of corticosteroids begun 12–24 hours prior to extubation appear beneficial for patients with a high likelihood of postextubation stridor.[30] Advantages of dexamethasone over methylprednisolone are the long half-life, which permits once-daily dosing, and fewer mineralocorticoid effects such as edema. Providing anticipatory guidance to the family members about what to expect may decrease their anxiety should the symptom occur.

Conclusion

Patients undergoing removal of respiratory life support are prone to distressing symptoms, including dyspnea and anxiety. Any plan for the discontinuation of therapy and goals of treatment must include management of potential symptoms and treatment for all distress.

References

1. Mazer M, Alligood CM, Wu Q. The infusion of opioids during terminal withdrawal of mechanical ventilation in the medical intensive care unit. *J Pain Symptom Manage*. 2011; 42(1): 44–51.

2. Rubenfeld GD, Crawford SW. Principles and practice of withdrawing life-sustaining treatment in the ICU. In: Curtis JR, Rubenfeld GD, eds. *Managing Death in the Intensive Care Unit*. New York, NY: Oxford University Press; 2001:127–47.

3. Hawryluck LA, Harvey WRC, Lemieux-Charles L, Singer PA. Consensus guidelines on analgesia and sedation in dying intensive care unit patients. *BMC Medical Ethics*. 2002; 3: 3. doi:10.1186/1472-6939-3-3.

4. Massachusetts General Hospital and Harvard Medical School. *Ventilator withdrawal guidelines*. American Association of Critical Care Nurses. Available at http://www.aacn.org/WD/Palliative/Content/tools-ventilatorwithdrawalguidelines.content?menu=Practice. Accessed October 23, 2016

5. Treece PD, Engelberg RA, Crowley L, et al. Evaluation of a standardized order form for withdrawal of life support in the intensive care unit. *Crit Care Med*. 2004; 32(7): 1141–8.

6. Curtis JR. Interventions to improve care during withdrawal of life-sustaining treatments. *J Palliat Med*. 2005; 8(Supp 1): S116–31.

7. Ward J. High-flow oxygen administration by nasal cannula for adult and perinatal patients. *Resp Care*. 2013; 58(1): 98–122.

8. Bazuaye EA, Stone TN, Corris PA, Gibson GJ. Variability of inspired oxygen concentration with nasal cannulas. *Thorax*. 1992; 47: 609.

9. Davidson PM, Johnson M. Update on the role of palliative oxygen. *Curr Opin Support Palliat Care*. 2011; 5: 87–91.

10. Campbell ML, Yarandi H, Dove-Medows E. Oxygen is non-beneficial for most patients who are near death. *J Pain Symptom Manag*. 2013; 45: 517–23.

11. Bausewein C, Booth S, Gysels M, Kuhnbach R, Higginson IJ. Effectiveness of a hand-held fan for breathlessness: a randomized phase II trial. *BMC Palliat Care*. 2010; 9: 22.

12. Peters SG, Holets SR, Gay PC. High-flow nasal cannula therapy in do-not-intubate patients with hypoxemic respiratory distress. *Resp Care*. 2013; 58: 597–600.

13. Lee JH, Rehder KJ, Williford L, Cheifetz IM, Turner DA. Use of high-flow nasal cannula in critically ill infants, children, and adults: a critical review of the literature. *Intens Care Med*. 2013; 39: 247–57.

14. Curtis JR, Cook DJ, Sinuff T, et al. Noninvasive positive pressure ventilation in critical and palliative care settings: understanding the goals of therapy. *Crit Care Med* 2007; 35(3): 932–9.

15. Nava S, Ferrer M, Esquinas A, et al. Palliative use of non-invasive ventilation in end-of-life patients with solid tumours: a randomized feasibility trial. *Lancet Oncol*. 2013; 14: 219–27.

16. International Consensus Conferences in Intensive Care Medicine. Noninvasive positive pressure ventilation in acute respiratory failure. *Am J Respir Crit Care Med*. 2001; 163(1): 283.

17. Edwards MJ. Opioids and benzodiazepines appear paradoxically to delay inevitable death after ventilator withdrawal. *J Palliat Care*. 2005; 21: 299–302.

18. Rady MY, Verheijde JL. The science and ethics of withdrawing mechanical positive pressure ventilator support in the terminally ill. *J Palliat Med*. 2013; 16(8): 828–30.

19. Park PK, Napolitano LM, Bartlett RH. Extracorporeal membrane oxygenation in adult acute respiratory distress syndrome. *Crit Care Clin*. 2011; 27: 627–46.

20. Extracorporeal Life Support Organization, *ELSO Guidelines for Cardiopulmonary Extracorporeal Life Support*. Available at http://www.elso.org/Portals/0/IGD/Archive/FileManager/6713186745cusersshyerdocumentselsoguidelinesforecprcases1.3.pdf November 2013: Version 1.3 Ann Arbor, MI. Accessed October 23, 2016.

21. Shekar K, Fraser JF, Smith MT, Roberts JA. Pharmacokinetic changes in patients receiving extracorporeal membrane oxygenation. *J Crit Care*. 2012; 27: 741.e9–741.e18

22. Grinnan DC, Swetz KM, Pinson J, Fairman P, Lyckholm LJ, Smith T. The end-of-life experience for a cohort of patients with pulmonary arterial hypertension. *J Palliat Care*. 2012; 15(10): 10651070.

23. McLaughlin VV, Palevsky HI. Parenteral and inhaled prostanoid therapy in the treatment of pulmonary arterial hypertension. *Clin Chest Med*. 2013; 34: 825–40.

24. Steinhauser KE, Clipp EC, McNeilly M, et al. In search of a good death: observations of patients, families, and providers. *Ann Intern Med*. 2000; 132: 825–32.

25. Steinhauser KE, Christakis NA, Clipp EC, et al. Factors considered important at the end of life by patients, family, physicians, and other care providers. *JAMA*. 2000; 284: 2476–82.

26. Campbell ML, Templin T, Walch J. A respiratory distress observation scale for patients unable to self-report dyspnea. *J Palliat Med*. 2010; 13(3): 285–90.

27. Campbell ML. How to withdraw mechanical ventilation: a systematic review of the literature. *AACN Adv Crit Care*. 2007; 18(4): 397–403

28. Campbell ML, Bizek KS, Thill M. Patient responses during rapid terminal weaning from mechanical ventilation: a prospective study. *Crit Care Med*. 1999; 27(1): 73–7.

29. Cheng KC, Hou CC, Huang HC. Intravenous injection of methylprednisolone reduces the incidence of postextubation stridor in intensive care unit patients. *Crit Care Med*. 2006; 34: 1345–50.

30. Khemani RG, Randolph A, Markovitz B. Corticosteroids for the prevention and treatment of post-extubation stridor in neonates, children and adults. *Cochrane Database of Systematic Reviews*. 2009, Issue 3. Art. No.: CD001000. doi: 10.1002/14651858.CD001000.pub3

Chapter 13

Palliative Sedation

Peg Nelson

Key Points

- Palliative sedation is an important therapy of last resort to relieve suffering in patients who have intractable pain and/or other symptoms.
- It requires knowledge of appropriate medications and an interdisciplinary approach.

Terms and Prevalence of Use

Palliative sedation may also be termed "terminal sedation," "sedation in patients with intractable symptoms," "sedation for intractable distress in the imminently dying," "end-of-life sedation," "total sedation," "controlled sedation," "palliative sedation therapy," and "proportionate sedation."[1]

Even though there is no universal definition of palliative sedation, there is agreement that it involves the monitored use of nonopioid medications to induce controlled sedation to the point of unconsciousness in a dying patient to relieve distress caused by otherwise uncontrolled pain and symptoms. Palliative sedation is different from procedural or conscious sedation, which is time-limited use of sedation to decrease awareness and discomfort during an anticipated painful procedure in a patient who is going to survive. Respite sedation is a time-limited use of sedative medications in dying patients with the goal of providing reprieve from distress and suffering for a period of time and then returning the patient to consciousness. See Box 13.1 for distinctions of palliative sedation.

It is important to understand and acknowledge the concerns of those who do not agree that the practice is morally acceptable. Objections include the fear that the practice leads to hastening death or euthanasia, thus violating the sanctity of life and the belief that God alone should choose when an individual dies. Similarly, the withdrawal of life support or withholding of other therapies, although legally permissible and ethically supported in medicine and nursing, is unacceptable within many individual's moral framework.[3] Thus, it is essential to understand the moral, legal, and ethical doctrines that support and challenge the use of palliative sedation while simultaneously initiating and participating in discussions about its use, with sensitivity to the concerns and perspectives of all: patients, families, and members of the healthcare team.

Box 13.1 Definitions of Types/Uses of Sedation

1. **Palliative sedation**: the controlled induction of sedation to the point of unconsciousness in a dying patient to relieve otherwise uncontrolled suffering; typically continued until the patient dies

2. **Procedural sedation**: the time-limited use of sedation to decrease awareness and pain during a medical procedure in a patient who is going to survive

3. **Respite sedation**: a time-limited use of palliative sedation medications in dying patients with the goal of giving respite from the suffering for a period of time and then returning the patient to consciousness.

Adapted from reference 2.

Creating a Model of Care for Palliative Sedation Therapy

To create a model of safe, effective, high-quality care, it is imperative to delineate the process of palliative sedation. Box 13.2 lists the five important aspects of palliative sedation policies and procedures.

Patient Eligibility

For the use of palliative sedation to be considered, the patient must have a terminal condition with imminent death anticipated; must have severe symptoms; and must be experiencing significant suffering, often described as intolerable, intractable, or refractory to aggressive standard palliative interventions. Imminent death is defined as a life expectancy of hours to days based on the person's current condition, the progression of disease, and the symptom constellation.[4]

The type of refractory patient suffering (physical vs. existential) for which palliative sedation therapy is considered should be clarified. The concepts of existential suffering and spiritual suffering are often interchangeable in the palliative literature.[5] A sense of purpose, freedom, and authenticity in life are fundamental existential attributes. The term "existential suffering" relates to the inability to find meaning, purpose, and fulfillment in one's life; a loss of dignity; fear of death; hopelessness; fear of being a burden

---

Box 13.2 Fundamental Elements of Patient Care for Palliative Sedation

- Patient eligibility
- Clinician/team member competence, involvement, and care
- Informed consent and decision-making (including the use of life-support nutrition, and hydration)
- Family involvement and care
- Medications and a procedure for palliative sedation

---

to others; and loneliness.[6-8] For some patients, such existential distress can be intolerable.

The use of palliative sedation for existential distress is controversial. It is the degree of the distress and the proximity of death that should be considered when determining whether to use palliative sedation. Refractory psychological distress must be distinguished from other treatable problems, such as depression, anxiety, delirium, other psychiatric illness, and family conflict. The American Medical Association's Opinion 2.201, Sedation to Unconsciousness in End-of-Life Care, recommends against the use of palliative sedation for existential distress.[9] Specific clinical guidelines pertinent to and applicable for the use of palliative sedation in the patient with existential suffering include:[10,11]

- All palliative treatments must be exhausted, including treatment for depression, delirium, anxiety, and any other contributing psychiatric illnesses or conditions.
- A psychological assessment by a skilled clinician should be completed.
- A spiritual assessment by a skilled clinician or member of the clergy should be done.
- A review of the case by interdisciplinary team members such as social workers, rehabilitation therapists
- A review of the case by various specialities, as appropriate, such as psychiatry, pain service; disease specialities such as pulmonary, gastroenterology, cardiology, neurology, oncology
- Informed consent should be obtained from the patient or surrogate decision-maker.

Consideration should be given to an initial trial of respite sedation, typically 24–48 hours. Respite palliative sedation has been found to be helpful for the patient, family, and healthcare team in re-evaluating the decision for and benefit of palliative sedation. There is general acceptance that when palliative sedation is considered, whether continuously or intermittently, there should be specific policies, procedures, and protocols for its use.[10,11] All treatment and diagnostic options for the previously discussed problems must be addressed adequately before palliative sedation is considered and provided. The decision to begin sedation is often difficult for clinicians, requiring thorough patient assessment and discussions with the patient, family, and other team members. See Box 13.3 for a template of a palliative sedation policy and procedure.

Clinician/Team Member Competence, Involvement, and Care

Interdisciplinary assessment determines the refractory nature of the symptoms. Key aspects include (1) ensuring that all standard treatments have been aggressively used and (2) determining that the symptom is truly refractory. Involving the social worker and/or the chaplain assists with the assessment and management of the patient's psychological and spiritual distress (which also affects his or her physical distress) and family and patient well-being and coping. The importance of addressing and treating the psychosocial distress

Box 13.3 Policy and Procedure for Palliative Sedation

a. Interdisciplinary assessment of the patient includes nursing, medical, social work, and chaplaincy providers.

b. The patient must be imminently dying.
   i. Life expectancy is hours to days.
   ii. There is a Do Not Resuscitate (DNR) order in place.

c. The patient has severe, intolerable pain and/or symptoms refractory to treatment.
   i. Aggressive palliative care management fails to provide relief.
   ii. Additional invasive/noninvasive treatment cannot provide relief.
   iii. Additional therapies are associated with excessive/unacceptable morbidity or are unlikely to provide relief within a reasonable time.
   iv. All palliative treatments must be exhausted, including treatment for depression, delirium, anxiety, and any other contributing psychiatric illnesses.
   v. Expert consultations from other specialties (i.e., psychiatry for delirium, pain service for pain syndromes, pulmonology for respiratory issues) offer no other alternatives.
   vi. A psychological assessment has been completed.
   vii. A spiritual assessment has been completed by a clinician or member of the clergy.

d. Trial of respite sedation may be considered before palliative sedation is provided.

Adapted from references 11 and 12.

that contributes to the patient's total pain expression cannot be overemphasized. A multidimensional approach is important to prevent, detect, and manage risk factors for intractable pain, including psychosocial distress, addictive behavior, and delirium in patients with terminal disease.

Collaboration with the interdisciplinary team not only validates the appropriateness of palliative sedation and facilitates the informed consent process but also reduces the emotional burden for the healthcare providers. During the process of palliative sedation, as well as before and after, there should be opportunities for team members to debrief, share concerns, and discuss personal distress.

In addition to ongoing team support, policies must also state how to handle conscientious objection by any member of the team to participating in palliative sedation and give procedures to transfer care to another available team member of equal competence while ensuring ongoing patient care. There should be mechanisms to discuss and resolve conflicts or concerns raised by anyone involved, along with consistent consultation with ethics committees and legal counsel. This promotes open communication within the organization.

Collaboration with other practitioners ensures that all reasonable treatment options to manage the distress have been exhausted and that the patient truly is near death. For safe and consistent practice, the palliative APRN should follow a palliative sedation policy or procedure. Information, education, and support for the health team about the process of decision-making and implementation of palliative sedation is imperative.

Informed Consent and Decision-Making

Informed consent requires the clinician to provide key information to the patient, so that the patient can weigh the risks and benefits of a procedure or treatment before reaching a voluntary decision about its use in his or her care.

If a patient is deemed to lack decision-making capacity, the surrogate decision-maker becomes the voice for the patient. Even if the patient is capable of making a decision, most protocols mention the importance of family members' being involved with the informed consent discussion along with the patient. Before palliative sedation is to be initiated, decisions regarding the use of life support, resuscitation, and artificial nutrition and hydration need to be determined separately from the decision for palliative sedation. Since palliative sedation is only used for the imminently dying, there should be a clear understanding that no attempt at cardiopulmonary resuscitation will occur, and the appropriate order (Do Not Resuscitate [DNR], Do Not Intubate [DNI], Do Not Attempt Resuscitation [DNAR]) will be in place before palliative sedation is provided. Other life-prolonging treatments, such as artificial nutrition and hydration, are typically also withdrawn before beginning palliative sedation, except for cases when respite sedation is being considered.

Family Involvement and Care

The palliative APRN should seek to elicit an understanding of the suffering of family members and provide careful, compassionate, and ongoing communication with them. Interdisciplinary care is critical at this time.

When patients are considering or undergoing palliative sedation, family distress may stem from many factors, including inability to interact with patient, anticipatory grief, disagreement or confusion regarding the use of sedation, perceptions that the use of sedation was precipitous or inappropriately delayed, and impressions that sedation hastened or actually caused the death or that death did not follow sedation as quickly as hoped.[13–15]

Communication and building trust are essential. If a patient or family members do not trust the healthcare team, conflict is likely to result.[16] Experts in palliative nursing stress the importance of deliberate, careful, and compassionate communication. Successful communication involves the principles listed in the companion volume to this book, *Advanced Practice Palliative Nursing* (2016), Chapter 40, Family Meetings, and Chapter 42, Navigating Ethical Discussions in Palliative Care.

Medications and Procedure of Sedation

The clinical, ethical, and legal decision-making for the use of palliative sedation includes determining the best type of sedative to use. The most common medications used for palliative sedation are barbiturates, benzodiazepines, and anesthetics. Patient assessment and clinical protocols developed by the interdisciplinary team, including pharmacists, guide drug selection, initial dosing, dose titration, and route of administration.[17] Opioids are not recommended as a sedative drug. However, they are used alongside sedatives as part of the management of pain or dyspnea.

Drug selection is based on the type of suffering that is present, current medications, response to past medications, the patient's medical problems, and the drug's efficacy, side-effect profile, and potential for success (Box 13.4). Although the intravenous route is preferred because it allows for quick titration and safety, subcutaneous administration is an acceptable alternative for some of the common medications.

Benzodiazepines are commonly used for palliative sedation; midazolam is often chosen due to its rapid onset of action and ease of titration.[18,19] The typical starting dose of midazolam is 2–5 mg given via an intravenous bolus (can be given subcutaneously) with a continuous infusion initiated at 1 mg per hour and titrated to achieve the level of sedation needed to provide relief.[20] Dosing may also be based on patient weight, with an initial intravenous bolus of 0.03–0.05 mg/kg and a continuous infusion that is initiated at 0.02–0.1 mg/kg/hour and titrated to effect.[21] Paradoxical agitation occasionally occurs with benzodiazepine use, especially in elderly patients with reduced liver function.[21] Reports also indicate that benzodiazepines sometimes fail to achieve adequate sedation.[22]

Barbiturates have been used for many years for palliative sedation.[23,24] Thiopental and pentobarbital have the quickest onsets of action and short durations, so they can be easily titrated. The starting dose for thiopental is an intravenous bolus of 5–7 mg/kg/hour and then 20–80 mg per hour as a continuous infusion. Pentobarbital is given as an intravenous bolus of 1–3 mg/kg, with a continuous infusion usually started at 1 mg/kg/hour.[23,24] Both thiopental and pentobarbital can be titrated to effect. Pentobarbital may offer antiemetic and anticonvulsant effects, making it more advantageous in patients at risk for vomiting and seizures.

Propofol (Diprivan) is considered an excellent agent for palliative sedation.[20] It can be used safely in patients who have renal or liver disease; it has an extremely short onset of action, duration of action, and half-life (shorter than

---

Box 13.4 Considerations for Palliative Sedation Medications

- The intractable pain or symptom being considered for palliative sedation
- History of medications used and their efficacy as well as current medications
- The patient's medical history and comorbid conditions
- Medication selection, including efficacy and rationale for potential for success
- Side-effect profile and potential interactions with current medications
- Best available route to administer medications appropriate to the setting of the patient. In the acute care setting, the intravenous route for palliative sedation is preferred due to the ability for quick titration and safety. However, subcutaneous administration is acceptable as an alternative in the acute care setting or the home.

the benzodiazepines and barbiturates); and it is very easy to titrate. It provides anxiolytic, antiemetic, antipruritic, anticonvulsant, antimyoclonic, and muscle relaxant effects.[20] Dosing for propofol is initially based on weight; a continuous infusion of 2.5–5 mcg/kg/minute can be increased by 2.5–5 mcg/kg/minute every hour to the desired level of sedation. During the infusion, the palliative APRN may also give bolus doses of propofol (2.5–5 mcg/kg) by intravenous push every 10 minutes as needed for rapid control of severe symptoms.[20]

Dexmedetomidine (Precedex) is a newer sedative agent that could be beneficial in palliative sedation, although it has not been studied extensively for this indication. It is an alpha-2 agonist that may induce unconsciousness without causing respiratory depression. The dosing range is typically 0.2–0.7 mcg/kg/hour. Loading or intravenous push doses are not needed. Avoiding a loading dose minimizes the risk of developing hypotension or bradycardia. The onset of effect of dexmedetomidine after beginning infusion is 5–10 minutes, with action lasting for approximately 60 minutes once the infusion is discontinued.[25,26]

Once the chosen medication is initiated, the level of sedation should be based on the predetermined patient goals and achievement of comfort. Sedation should not be increased unless the patient shows signs of distress, such as restlessness, grimacing, or findings that could reasonably be interpreted as evidence of suffering (including tachypnea and tachycardia). Otherwise, increasing sedation without an overt clinical indication might imply the clinician is intending to hasten death and would ostensibly cross the line between palliative sedation and physician-assisted suicide or euthanasia.[27] Current assessment tools to monitor conscious sedation in hospitals are not appropriate for the dying patient. The level of sedation needed varies with each patient and is based on the achievement of comfort and predetermined goals.

Conclusion

Although palliative sedation is used only when patients experience the most extreme distress, it is a therapy that is a core competency of the palliative APRN and the palliative care team. A policy and procedure should be developed using the resources of an organization, including the pharmacotherapeutics committee, the ethics committee, and clinical practice committee. Guidelines should include the ethics that support palliative sedation, medications, communication, and emotional and legal support. When palliative sedation is considered, it is an interdisciplinary team process that includes education and support for both the palliative care team members and the health team.

References

1. Sterckx S, Raus K, Mortier F, eds. *Continuous Sedation at End of Life—Ethical, Clinical and Legal Perspectives*. Cambridge, UK: Cambridge University Press; 2013:30.

2. Quill TE, Miller FG. Physician-assisted death. In: Quill TE, Miller FG eds. *Palliative Care and Ethics*. New York, NY: Oxford University Press; 2014:247.

3. Billings JA. Palliative sedation. In: Quill TE, Miller FG, eds. *Palliative Care and Ethics*. New York, NY: Oxford University Press; 2014: 209–30.

4. Cowan JD, Walsh D. Terminal sedation in palliative medicine—definition and review of the literature. *Support Care Cancer*. 2001; 9: 403–7.

5. Boston P, Bruce A, Schreiber R. Existential suffering n the palliative care setting; An integrated literature review. *J Pain Symptom Manage*. 2011; 41(3): 604–18.

6. Okon T. Palliative care review: spiritual, religious and existential aspects of palliative care. *J Palliat Med*. 2005; 8: 392–411.

7. Morita T, Tsunoda J, Satoshi I, Chihara S. An exploratory factor analysis of existential suffering in the Japanese terminally ill patients. *Psychooncology*. 2000; 9: 164–8.

8. McSherry W, Cash K. The language of spirituality: an emerging taxonomy. *Intl J Nurs Stud*. 2004; 41: 151–61.

9. American Association of Hospice and Palliative Medicine (Board of Directors). *Advisory Brief: Guidance on Responding to Requests for Physician-Assisted Dying*. December 2015. Available at http://aahpm.org/positions/padbrief. Accessed October 23, 2016.

10. Rousseau PC. Palliative sedation: a brief review of ethical validity and clinical experience. *Mayo Clin Proc*. 2000; 75: 1064–9.

11. Rousseau P. Existential suffering and palliative sedation: a brief commentary with a proposal for clinical guidelines. *Am J Hosp Palliat Care*. 2001; 18(3): 151–3.

12. Cherny NI, Portenoy RK. Sedation in the management of refractory symptoms: guidelines for evaluation and treatment. *J Palliat Care*. 1994; 10: 31–8.

13. Higgins PC, Altillo T. Palliative sedation: an essential place for clinical excellence. *J Social Work End Life Palliat Care*. 2007; 3(4): 3–30.

14. Brajtman S, The impact on the family of terminal restlessness and its management. *Palliat Med*. 2003; 17(5): 454–60.

15. Morita T, Ikenaga M, Adachi I, et al. Concerns of family members of patients receiving palliative sedation therapy. *Support Care Cancer*. 2004; 12 (12): 885–9.

16. Caplan AL. Odds and ends: trust and the debate over medical futility. *Ann Intern Med*. 1996; 125: 688–9.

17. Schildmann MS, Schildmann MA. Palliative sedation therapy: a systemic literature review and critical appraisal of available guidance on indication and decision-making. *J Palliat Med*. 2014; 17(5): 601–11.

18. Levy MH, Cohen SD. Sedation for the relief of refractory symptoms in the imminently dying: a fine intentional line. *Semin Oncol*. 2005; 32: 237–46.

19. Salacz M, Weissman DE. Fast Facts and Concepts #107 *Controlled sedation for refractory suffering—part II*. 2015. Palliative Care Network of Wisconsin. Available at http://www.mypcnow.org/blank-m3r0z. Accessed October 23, 2016.

20. Krakauer EL, Quinn TE. Sedation in palliative medicine. In: Hanks G, Cherny N, Christakis NA, Fallon M, Kaasa S, Portenoy RK, eds. *Oxford Textbook of Palliative Medicine*. 4th ed. New York, NY: Oxford University Press; 2011:1560–7.

21. Shafer A. Complications of sedation with midazolam in the intensive care unit and a comparison with other sedative regimens. *Crit Care Med*. 1998; 26: 947–56.

22. Cheng C, Roemer-Becuwe C, Pereira J. When midazolam fails. *J Pain Symptom Manage*. 2002; 23: 256–65.

23. Truog RD, Berda CB, Mitchell C, Grier HE. Barbiturates in the care of the terminally ill. *N Engl J Med*. 1992; 327: 1678–82.

24. Greene WR, Davis WH. Titrated intravenous barbiturates in the control of symptoms in patients with terminal cancer. *South Med J* 1991; 84: 332–7.

25. Jackson KC, Paul W, Fine PG. Dexmedetomidine: a novel analgesic with palliative medicine potential. *J Pain Palliat Care Pharmacol*. 2006; 20:23–7.

26. Prommer E. Dexmedetomidine: does it have potential in palliative medicine? *J Hosp Palliat Care*. 2011; 28: 276–83.

27. Alpers A, Lo B. The Supreme Court addresses physician-assisted suicide. Can its rulings improve palliative care? *Arch Family Med*. 1999; 8(3): 200–5.

Chapter 14

Pediatric Palliative Care Across the Continuum

Vanessa Battista and Gina Santucci

Key Points

- Pediatric palliative care (PPC) is interdisciplinary, family-centered care that focuses on a child's and family's quality of life through the prevention and relief of suffering along a physical, psychological, emotional, spiritual, and social continuum. Care is provided on both an inpatient and outpatient basis.
- Principles for assessing and managing pain in children are unique and must take into account the child's developmental, cognitive, and biological factors.
- A growing number of families choose to have their children die at home, necessitating more home-based PPC and hospice services. A variety of factors must be considered when caring for children and families in their home setting.

Child–Family Unit

Parents, family members, siblings, and the child all suffer throughout the course of an illness, and although this may manifest differently, each person's suffering somehow affects the others.[1] Schedules and daily family routines are interrupted, and parents may struggle to find enough time and energy to spend with each other and the ill child's siblings to transport them to their after-school activities or to attend events at school.

Siblings

Although there is little published evidence to support this hypothesis, it is well-recognized that siblings experience a significant amount of stress when their brothers or sisters face life-threatening illness. Parents and other caregivers, including healthcare providers, must pay close attention to signs and symptoms of sibling distress. Siblings can have elevated rates of anxiety and depression, symptoms of post-traumatic stress disorder, decreased participation in activities, difficulties in school, lower cognitive development scores, and overall ratings of poor/diminished quality of life.[2] Supports are crucial for siblings, such as school, community, and camp programs, as well as professional counseling and/or support group services that may be available either at the hospital or through an outpatient setting.[3]

Designating a "special person," such as a friend or relative who can take responsibility for each sibling specifically, may be helpful, so that siblings get extra attention. Parents and caretakers may also find it helpful to dedicate a specific time of day to spend with siblings and to maintain their normal routine as much as possible.[3]

Extended Family

Everyone considered part of a child's family, including grandparents, aunts and uncles, cousins, and friends, can be affected when a child has a life-threatening illness. Whether a child's illness lasts for a short time or extends over many years, the ramifications of life with an ill child can have lasting effects on marriages, partnerships, and relationships; cause stress and physical and/or mental health problems; affect finances and/or employment status; create social isolation or disengagement from peer-related activities; and foster a sense of loss, concern for the future, and grief.[4] Specific family members may also have particular needs or concerns that warrant attention. Grandparents are often very involved in a child's care and may report feeling helpless because they not only are unable to protect their grandchild from illness, but also cannot protect their own child, the parent, from the pain and suffering he or she is experiencing.

Evidence shows that clinicians' attention to the needs of family members can enhance their resiliency.[4] Overall, families are amazingly resilient, but they may need guidance in figuring out new roles and ways in which they can support each other since everyone copes in his or her own unique way.

Community and School

Nearly all families belong to at least one type of community, and children are often at the epicenter of community-based activities. Whether it is through their school, place of worship, neighborhood, sports team, or other recreational activity (e.g., Girl Scouts or Boy Scouts), families find a sense of belonging with others in which camaraderie and relationships form. Similar to the effects on extended family, when a child becomes ill, the whole community may also feel the consequences of the illness. Community members may show concern and play a tremendous role in providing support to the child and family.

Children living with chronic or life-threatening illnesses often receive much of their care during the school day. Physical, emotional, or developmental challenges may necessitate attendance at a specialized school with an individualized education plan and appropriate therapeutic services in place. It is important and helpful to include school-based teams in decision-making, to keep them informed of decisions that are made, and to have palliative care conversations in schools.[5,6]

Child's View of Illness and Death

Every child will have his or her personalized integration of his or her illness experience. Garnering a sense from a child about his or her illness interpretation is not always an easy task, however. Children express themselves in different ways; some use words, some draw pictures, some engage in play, some use body language and behavior, and some don't speak at all.

Every child has a unique perspective on his or her illness experience depending on his or her developmental stage.[7] In particular, different developmental tasks influence how children perceive and cope with illness and possible death. Table 14.1 summarizes children's developmental stages and perceptions of death in each stage.

Goals of Care, Limitations of Care, and Decision-Making

Code Status Discussions

Despite advances in medical technology, the number of children living with life-threatening illness is on the rise. Families frequently are faced with difficult decisions about whether to forgo life-sustaining medical treatment and/or to elect that Do Not Attempt Resuscitation (DNAR), Do Not Resuscitate (DNR), or Do Not Intubate (DNI) orders be placed for their children. The nomenclature around this topic has changed in recent years: the terms, Do Not Attempt Resuscitation and Allow Natural Death (AND), are being used increasingly in more organizations instead of DNR. The code status DNAR signifies that not all attempts at resuscitation will be successful. The code status AND is thought to be more acceptable from a family standpoint, signifying as it does death as the result of natural disease progression.[10] However, for some families of children, there may be no natural death because a child is not supposed to die before a parent.

Predicting outcomes for children living with life-threatening illness is a complex and often difficult task. Thus, helping children, when chronologically and developmentally appropriate, and their families decide whether to limit interventions is often a multifaceted task. A good approach to deciding about limitations of care may include discussions with families regarding when "cardiopulmonary resuscitation (CPR) or other medical and procedural interventions may seriously impair the quality of life"[11] or when it may interfere with the ability or desire to achieve important life goals.[11] Most important, however, is to recognize that decisions about resuscitation status are usually the result of several discussions between providers and family members about their goals of care for their children and family. The work of the team or the teams involved in these discussions then becomes to help families understand what interventions may or may not be beneficial to their children (e.g., chest compressions, intubation) and ways in which they can "secure for the incurable child a death filled with dignity and free from excessive suffering and treatment-related morbidity."[11]

Decision-Making and Honoring Wishes

Decisions about what interventions to choose are seldom black-and-white. Having tools to guide decision-making and conversations about goals of care are extremely helpful. It is also paramount to include children in age- and developmentally-appropriate conversations regarding their goals. Some children may

Table 14.1 Developmental Stages and Perceptions of Death

Age	Basic Conflict	View of Death	Suggestions
Birth–18 months	Trust vs. mistrust	• No sense of finality and is viewed as continuous with life • Reactive to stress	• Use simple physical communication and provide comforting and nurturing care.
Early childhood (2–3 years)	Autonomy vs. shame and doubt	• Death is seen as reversible and not final • May feel that death is a punishment • May feel responsible for death	• Expect regression, clinging, or aggressive behavior. • Encourage expression, as the child may be concerned about family function after he or she dies. • Use honest and clear language to explain death and dying.
Preschool (3–5 years)	Initiative vs. guilt	• Death continues to be understood as temporary • May have a literal understanding of death and will respond with curiosity and questioning	• Continue to use open communication with clear language. • Encourage questions about death and dying.
School age (6–11 years)	Industry vs. inferiority	• Death is understood as permanent and that the body ceases to function, with heart and respirations stopping • May feel responsible and guilty for the illness • May have spiritual ideas about afterlife • May not want to discuss feelings	• Reassure the child that death is not his or her fault. • Strive to maintain as normal a structure as possible. • Include the child in afterlife plans (funeral planning, last wishes).
Adolescence (12–18 years)	Identity vs. role confusion	• Understands the finality of death and may develop a mature understanding of death • May try to take responsibility for adult concerns within the family (such as finances and caretaking) • Feelings of anger may be present	• Allow time for reflection. • Listen to concerns and questions. • Support efforts for autonomy and control.

Adapted from references 8 and 9; printed in reference 7.

explicitly express their wishes regarding their end-of-life and/or resuscitation status; other children may not want to address these topics. In some cases, children may feel more comfortable talking with healthcare providers than talking with their family. They may fear disappointing their family if they choose not to pursue particular interventions. At other times, children and their parents/guardians may disagree about what the goals of care should be and/or what particular interventions they should choose to receive. Helpful documents include *My Wishes* (for young children), *Voicing My Choices* (for adolescents), and *Five Wishes* (for adults), published by Aging with Dignity and available at www.agingwithdignity.org.

Cardiac Disorders

Heart failure in children is usually seen in those diagnosed with either congenital heart defects or cardiomyopathies; a smaller number will have conditions that directly affect the myocardium (Box 14.1). Children who have surgical palliation of their congenital heart disease are also at risk for developing heart failure. The diagnosis of heart failure is based on several clinical factors, including whether the child has an underlying cardiac defect or a weakened heart muscle.

Children with congenital heart disease often live with increased morbidity and may require frequent hospital stays to manage their complex needs. See the companion volume to this book, *Advanced Practice Palliative Nursing* (2016), Chapter 58: Pediatric Palliative Care Across the Continuum for a complete discussion. Regardless of the etiology, children with end-stage heart failure may be cared for in a variety of settings, including at home, in a community-based hospice, or in an inpatient setting such as the ICU. The location of care depends on the goals of care, the family's ability to provide care at home, available resources, and, ultimately, where the dying child's and family's needs can be met. Although many children born with congenital heart disease do well, some will require multiple surgeries and frequent

---

Box 14.1 Congenital Heart Defects

- Transposition of great arteries
- Tetralogy of Fallot
- Tricuspid or pulmonary atresia
- Ebstein's anomaly
- Hypoplastic left heart syndrome
- Truncus arteriosus
- Double outlet right ventricle
- Heterotaxy
- Atrial and ventricular septal defects
- Total or partial anomalous pulmonary venous return

From Center for Disiease Control and Prevention. Specific Congential Heart Defects. Last updated 2015. http://www.cdc.gov/ncbddd/heartdefects/specificdefects.html. Accessed October 23, 2016.

Table 14.2 Medication Guidelines for Heart Failure

	Options	Notes
Preload reduction	Furosemide (PO, IV)	Loop diuretic. Indomethacin may reduce effects.
	Hydrochlorothiazide (PO)	Thiazide diuretic. Use with caution in renal disease.
	Bumetanide (PO, IV)	Loop diuretic. Contraindicated in anuria or azotemia.
Afterload reduction	Captopril (PO)	Angiotensin-converting enzyme inhibitor (ACEI). Use caution in bilateral renal stenosis, renal impairment.
	Enalapril (PO)	ACE. Use caution in bilateral renal stenosis, renal impairment.
	Alprostadil (IV)	Maintains patency of ductus arteriosus. Important in ductal dependent defects.
Improve contractility	Digoxin (PO/IV)	Slows ventricular rate. Contraindicated in AV block.
	Dopamine (IV)	Correct hypovolemia prior to starting.
	Milrinone (IV)	Fewer cardiovascular side effects than other medications

Data from Medications Used to Treat Heart Failure http://www.heart.org/HEARTORG/Conditions/HeartFailure/PreventionTreatmentofHeartFailure/Heart-Failure-Medications_UCM_306342_Article.jsp; and 2013 ACCF/AHA Guideline for the Management of Heart Failure http://circ.ahajournals.org/content/128/16/e240.extract; Accessed October 23, 2016.

hospital admissions for ongoing care. Eventually, the involvement of a PPC team can provide support for children, siblings, and parents; assist with symptom management and decision-making; and, ultimately, prepare the family for care at the end of life.

Most medications used to manage heart failure are available either orally or intravenously (Table 14.2) and should be initiated and managed by a provider with cardiology expertise.

Technical support, such as extracorporeal membrane oxygenation (ECMO) or a ventricular assist device (VAD), may be an option for some children depending on the family's goals of care.[12] Some children in heart failure who are waiting for a transplant may require ECMO or a VAD as a bridge to heart transplantation.[13] However, for children who are not candidates for a heart transplant, implantation of a VAD may provide long-term support in certain settings. In PPC, using a VAD as "destination therapy" is becoming an option in certain centers.[14] The decision to use ECMO or a VAD should not be considered in juxtaposition with the goals of palliative care. Healthcare providers need to balance interventions that may offer some benefit with those that clearly do not. Once a family has made the decision to pursue advanced technologies, it becomes the healthcare provider's responsibility to manage pain, support the family, and provide guidance regarding withdrawal of support, when necessary. Advance planning for children with congenital heart disease should include not only discussions about resuscitation and DNAR but also when the use of advanced technologies like ECMO, VAD, and other invasive procedures would be appropriate and when they would not.[15]

Cystic Fibrosis

Cystic fibrosis is an autosomal recessive genetic disorder caused by a mutation of the cystic fibrosis transmembrane conductance regulator (CFTR) gene. It is the second most common childhood genetic disorder, with approximately 30,000 people living with the disease in North America.[16] Cystic fibrosis occurs in 1 in 3,700 live births, and every year approximately 1,000 patients are newly diagnosed.[17] This progressive, life-threatening disease affects multiple organ systems; chronic respiratory infections, inflammation, and pulmonary decline are the primary causes of morbidity and mortality.[18] Other causes of illness and decline are poor growth, malabsorption, pancreatic insufficiency, diabetes mellitus, hemolytic anemia, and hepatic biliary disease.[19] Currently, there is no cure, but with improvements in technology, aggressive medical management, and supportive care, many children are living into early adulthood, albeit with an increase in morbidity. For certain children with advanced disease, lung transplantation may be an option.

From the time of diagnosis, children with cystic fibrosis must endure multiple therapies and frequent hospital stays to manage disease exacerbations. The decision of whether to integrate a palliative approach to care can be challenging. (Box 14.2).

Managing progressive dyspnea, fatigue, and pain in cystic fibrosis, especially at the end of life, can be challenging. Pain and discomfort are intensified by inflammation of the pleura, cough, rib fractures, and the need for aggressive respiratory treatments. Overwhelmingly, evidence supports the benefits of using small doses of opioids to treat dyspnea and

---

Box 14.2 The Collaborative Benefit of Palliative Care Services in Children with Cystic Fibrosis

- Prior to diagnosis, help the primary care team create a supportive approach for infants who screen positive for the disease.
- Collaborate with the team to develop strategies to reduce parental grief when given the news that their child has a life-threatening disease.
- Support the team during admissions, provide strategies to decrease stress, and offer help with pain and symptom management as needed.
- As the disease progresses, collaborate with the team and family on treating bothersome pain and symptoms, answering difficult questions, addressing the "what-ifs" and use of aggressive technologies, developing approaches to facilitate discussions related to transplantation, providing support to siblings, and suggesting care settings, including hospice.
- Develop a plan to address support for family and medical providers at the time of death, including community services to provide ongoing bereavement services.

Adapted from reference 20.

benzodiazepines to treat associated anxiety.[21] Some clinicians and family members may fear that using opioids may shorten the child's life (i.e., hasten death) or that the child will become addicted to them. It is the role of the PPC team to help clinicians and families overcome such fears and misconceptions about opioid use. For children with cystic fibrosis, opioids and nonpharmacologic measures may be the only options to palliate progressive symptoms at the end of life. Nonpharmacologic measures, such as noninvasive positive pressure ventilation (NIPPV), supplemental oxygen, and use of a fan, may also provide relief of dyspnea. PPC teams, in collaboration with cystic fibrosis teams, can provide the interdisciplinary support that is needed when caring for children with progressive, chronic, life-threatening conditions.

Neoplasms

The overall 5-year survival rate for children with some forms of cancer is currently 80–85%. In acute lymphoblastic leukemia, non-Hodgkin's lymphoma, and Wilms tumor, this number can exceed 90%.[22] Until recently, children diagnosed with brain tumors had survival rates of less than 50%, and although there are still uniformly fatal brain tumors, interventions like surgery, chemotherapy, and radiation have increased survival rates to above 75%.[23]

Brain and spinal tumors account for 20% of all pediatric cancers and are the most common type of solid tumors in children. Treatment usually consists of a combination of surgery, chemotherapy, and radiation. Radiation is usually delayed in children under the age of 5 years to preserve neurocognition in the developing brain. Tumor location, cell biology, and metastases will determine what treatments will be offered. Not all brain tumors are malignant, but even nonmalignant ones can be life-threatening due to their location, their impact on the surrounding tissue, and their potential to cause increased intracranial pressure. Clinical symptoms depend on the site of involvement and may include headaches, seizures, loss of vision, hemiparesis, ataxia, nerve palsy, macrocephaly in infants, loss of developmental milestones, and vomiting.[24] Depending on tumor location, endocrine disorders such as diabetes insipidus can occur. Treatments can cause personality changes, memory loss, and hormonal dysfunction.

Children with brain tumors require a multidisciplinary approach, and PPC should be introduced as soon as possible to provide ongoing psychosocial support and pain and symptom management. Medications and treatments to cure or palliate can become a source of additional pain, worsening symptoms, and longer hospital stays. Many children require central lines, ventricular-peritoneal shunts, frequent imaging, high-dose corticosteroids, radiation, and chemotherapy. Acute changes in neurological function may require ICU interventions, such as externalization of shunts, mechanical ventilation, and repeat surgeries. When cure is not possible, treatments become a balance of preserving function, maximizing quality of life, and minimizing deficits. PPC teams can facilitate communication, help with decisions regarding aggressive interventions, acknowledge uncertainty, and offer a space for meaningful conversations regarding prognosis.[25]

Spinal Muscular Atrophy

Spinal muscular atrophy (SMA) is an incurable autosomal recessive disorder that causes generalized weakness and atrophy of the voluntary muscles. It is classified into six clinical types; in this chapter, we focus on type 1 (Werdnig-Hoffman disease). SMA type 1 is considered a severe form of the disease and occurs in 4.1 per 100,000 live births.[26] Clinical features are hypotonia, symmetrical weakness, poor head control, weak cry and cough, and absent deep tendon reflexes. Cognition and sensation are not affected. SMA is a progressive disease that eventually affects the diaphragm and all voluntary muscles.[27] Hallmark clinical findings include the inability to clear secretions, hypoventilation during sleep, underdeveloped respiratory muscles, and frequent infections that worsen the child's overall weakness.[27] The risk for aspiration, pneumonia, and rapid respiratory decline is considerable, and often these children will have a natural death before 24 months if mechanical ventilation is not pursued. Given the early disease onset, severity of illness, and potential life-threatening complications, involvement of the PPC team is often recommended at the time of diagnosis.

Pain Management Considerations

The same guiding principles used for managing pain in adults can be applied to children, with a few caveats. See the companion volume to this book, *Advanced Practice Palliative Nursing* (2016), Chapter 23: Pain, for a thorough description of medications, pharmokinetics, and dosing. The child's developmental age, cognitive ability, weight, the impact of pain on the child and family, and the maturity of the patient's renal and hepatic systems all affect pediatric pain assessment, management, and appropriate medication use. PPC teams, in consultation with the primary team caring for the child, should develop plans that partner with children and parents. A good pain management plan includes a thorough assessment using appropriate tools, a clarification of the goals of treatment, a description of expected side effects, a discussion of how increased pain will be addressed, and, the incorporation of nonpharmacologic therapies (e.g., distraction, relaxation techniques, acupuncture, guided imagery, play).[28]

Special attention must be given to nonverbal children and those with cognitive or developmental disabilities. This is a vulnerable group, and their inability to self-report pain can result in erroneous and inappropriate management.[29] Children with advanced disease deserve optimal pain control. For children who are at the end of life, managing pain and other bothersome symptoms must be a priority. No one wants to see children suffer needlessly in pain, yet many children with advanced illness do not have adequate pain control[30] (Table 14.3).

The World Health Organization (WHO) and the American Academy of Pediatrics offer clear guidelines on how to initiate and escalate pain management in children. There is no standard dosing for opioids; rather, "the right dose is the dose that works." For children who have been exposed to opioids in the past, start with the drug and dose that were previously safe and effective. For those who are opioid naïve, start with a low dose based on weight and general health and titrate upward, balancing analgesia and sedation or other adverse effects.

Table 14.3 Pain Behaviors in Children	
Infancy (1–12 months)	Inconsolability
	Feeding/sleeping difficulty
	Grimacing
	Change in activity level
	High-pitched cry
	Frequent yawning
	Tachycardia/tachypnea
Toddler (1–4 years)	Lost interest in play
	Moaning
	Irritability
	Loss of appetite
	Difficulty sleeping or excessive sleeping
	Overly clingy
	Guarding
School-age and adolescent (5–17 years)	Change in activity level
	Overly quiet or subdued
	Irritable or angry
	Mismatched cues
	Difficulty sleeping

Adapted from reference 30.

Patient-controlled analgesia (PCA) involves an infusion pump that can be programmed to deliver medications at continuous prescribed doses and also can allow the patient (or parent) to deliver boluses of medication. Children as young as 3 or 4 years can be taught how to "press the button" to deliver pain medications. PCA should be considered when (1) pain is not controlled on increasing doses of oral or transdermal medication, (2) pain is not controlled on adequate doses of around-the-clock intravenous opioids, (3) pain is expected to escalate quickly, (4) routine care causes significant pain and may require additional dosing before activity, and (5) the child wants more control or the provider wants to give the child more control over the pain. The two main disadvantages of PCA are a child's unwillingness to use it and the need for intravenous or subcutaneous access. Morphine and hydromorphone are the common PCA opioids utilized, although circumstances may necessitate the use of fentanyl. Depending on the goals of care and resuscitation status, a bag-valve mask, supplemental oxygen, and continuous pulse oximetry may be needed for the first 24 hours on PCA and with subsequent dose increases.

Post-Acute Care

Considerations for Going Home

An increasing number of families are choosing to keep their children at home for the duration of their disease and, ultimately, their death. This is a very personal choice for families and is based on a variety of factors, such as available resources and support, who lives at home, and the family's past experiences with death. As with other decisions, families must be assured that there is no "right or wrong" choice about keeping the child in the hospital or at home. As with any comprehensive PPC plan, a home care plan should include careful assessment of the child's physical needs and emotional symptoms and the child's and family's developmental level and ability to complete developmental tasks. Practical factors, such as finances, living situation, social support, and religious or spiritual/existential beliefs and practices, should be considered.[31] The focus is to ensure that families have their physical, emotional, and social needs met, whether they choose to remain in the hospital or transition to home.

Hospice Care

Many hospices have nurses and other team members, such as social workers and chaplains, who are dedicated to providing high-quality hospice care for children and their families. It is helpful to identify dedicated pediatric hospice partners in the community. In many instances, the inpatient PPC team will direct the care for children at home with hospice, working directly with hospice providers to adjust medications and care plans to maintain children's comfort and support families while at home. Some hospices have inpatient units where children can go, and it is helpful to identify what resources are available for families in different geographic areas served by the PPC team.

Concurrent Care

On March 23, 2010, the federal government enacted the "concurrent care for children" provision in Section 2302 of the Patient Protection and Affordable Health Care Act (PPACA).[32] This provision allows children with state Medicaid or Children's Health Insurance Programs (CHIP) to receive hospice care while still receiving curative treatment (i.e., blood products, antibiotics, infusions, lab tests) and home nursing services.

Care While at Home

Aside from resources like hospice and home health, there are several practical aspects that should be considered when providing care for a child at home. It is extremely important to consider who will manage pain and other symptoms in the home and to have a plan in place for medication management. Often this will be managed by a hospice and/or home care nurse in the home, but parents may also be involved in dosing and providing medications. It is also important to make sure that medications are kept in a safe place and are locked up, if necessary. A pain and symptom management plan should be communicated to the care providers (i.e., hospice, home care, and family members) to ensure that the child is both safe and comfortable.

Care at the Time of Death and Beyond

Many families describe the death of their children at home as a sacred and beautiful event. Therefore, everything possible must be done to allow families this experience and to keep things calm. All necessary medications and other supplies, such as dark towels for potential bleeding, should be in the home in advance. Alternative routes for medication delivery should also be considered. Some families may want private time with their children prior to, surrounding, and following the time of death. Other families may request that family members and clinical providers be present. It is helpful to discuss this in advance and to have a plan in place for what will occur at the time surrounding the child's death. Families may have specific cultural and/or spiritual customs and rituals at the time of death, and these practices should be honored and respected. Families may want photos taken of their children and keepsakes created, such as hand molds and prints, and they may choose to have siblings and other family members participate in creating these items. Families may participate in the physical care of the child at the time of death, such as bathing and dressing, and this option should be given to families.

Conclusion

PPC is an emerging and multifactorial area of healthcare that is on the rise as increasing attention is being given to children living with life-threatening illnesses and their need for optimal quality of life and pain and symptom management. PPC is family-centered care by nature and focuses on addressing the needs of children living with life-threatening illness as well as the needs of their family and community members. PPC is often initiated as the goals of care shift from a focus on cure to a focus on optimizing quality of life, and a properly trained team of interdisciplinary professionals is necessary to deliver this type of care, both in the hospital and at home.

References

1. Roets L, Rowe-Rowe N, Nel R. Family-centered care in the paediatric intensive care unit. *J Nurs Manag*. 2012; 20(5): 624–30.

2. Muriel AC, Case C, Sourkes B. Children's voices: the experience of patients and their siblings. In: Hinds PS, Sourkes BM, Wolfe J, eds. *Textbook of Interdisciplinary Pediatric Palliative Care*. Philadelphia, PA: Saunders, 2011:18–29.

3. Bergstraesser E. Pediatric palliative care—when quality of life becomes the main focus of treatment. *Eur J Pediatr*. 2013; 172(2): 139–50.

4. Jone B, Contro N, Koch KK. The duty of the physician to care for the family in pediatric palliative care: context, communication, and caring. *Pediatrics*. 2014; 133(S1): S8–15.

5. Levetown M. Communicating with children and families: from everyday interactions to skill in conveying distressing information. *Pediatrics*. 2008; 121(5): e1441–60.

6. Ross ME, Hicks J, Furman WL. Preschool as palliative care. *J Clin Oncol*. 2008; 26(22): 3797–9.

7. Mandac C, Battista V. Contributions of palliative care to pediatric patient care. *Semin Oncol Nurs*. 2014; 30(4): 1–15.

8. Vern-Gross T. Establishing communication within the field of pediatric oncology: a palliative care approach. *Curr Probl Cancer*. 2011; 35(6): 337–50.

9. Foster TL, Bell CJ, Gilmer MJ. Symptom management of spiritual suffering in pediatric palliative care. *J Hosp Palliat Nurs*. 2012; 14(2): 109–15.

10. World Health Organization. *WHO Definiton of Palliative Care*. Available at www.worldhealthorganization.com and http://www.who.int/cancer/palliative/definition/en/. Accessed October 23, 2016.

11. Baker JN. Resuscitation. In: Hinds PS, Sourkes BM, Wolfe J, eds. *Textbook of Interdisciplinary Pediatric Palliative Care*. Philadelphia, PA: Saunders; 2011:199–203.

12. Fynn-Thompson F, Almond C. Pediatric assisted ventricular devices. *Pediatr Cardiol*. 2007; 28(2): 149–55.

13. De Rita F, Hasan A, Haynes S, et al. Mechanical cardiac support in children with congenital heart disease with intention to bridge to heart transplantation. *Eur J Cardiothorac Surg*. 2014; 46(4): 656–62.

14. Drakos SG, Charitos EI, Nanas SN, et al. Ventricular assist device for treatment of chronic heart failure. *Expert Rev Cardiovasc Ther*. 2007; 5(3): 571–84.

15. Blume E, Green A. Advanced heart disease. In: Hinds PS, Sourkes BM, Wolfe J, eds. *Textbook of Interdisciplinary Pediatric Palliative Care*. Philadelphia, PA: Saunders; 2011:428–37.

16. O'Sullivan BP, Freedman SD. Cystic fibrosis. *Lancet*. 2009; 373(9678): 1891–904.

17. American Lung Association. *State of Lung Disease in Diverse Communities*. Available at http://www.lung.org/assets/documents/publications/solddc-chapters/cf.pdf. Accessed October 23, 2016.

18. Bonfield TL, Panuska JR, Konstan MW, et al. Inflammatory cytokines in cystic fibrosis lungs. *Am J Respir Crit Care Med*. 1995; 152(6): 2111–8.

19. US National Library of Medicine. Genetic Home Reference. *Cystic fibrosis*. Available at http://ghr.nlm.nih.gov/condition/cystic-fibrosis. Prepared September 2014. Accessed October 23, 2016.

20. Pian P, Goggin J. Cystic fibrosis. In: Ferguson-Hendricks V, ed. *Palliative Care for Pediatric Life-Limiting Conditions*. Pittsburgh, PA: Hospice and Palliative Care Association; 2014:83–112.

21. Bourke SJ, Doe SJ, Gascoigne AD, et al. An integrated model of provision of palliative care to patients with cystic fibrosis. *Palliat Med*. 2009; 23(6): 512–7.

22. LaFond D, Rood B, Jacobs S, et al. Integration of therapeutic and palliative care in pediatric oncology. In: Hinds PS, Sourkes BM, Wolfe J, eds. *Textbook of Interdisciplinary Pediatric Palliative Care*. Philadelphia, PA: Saunders; 2011:460–9.

23. National Cancer Institute. Surveillence, Epidimiology, and End Results Program. *Childhood Cancer: SEER Cancer Statistics Review*. Updated September 16, 2016. Available at http://seer.cancer.gov/csr/1975_2013/results_merged/sect_29_childhood_cancer_iccc.pdf#search=childhood+cancer. Accessed October 23, 2016.

24. Arland LC, Hendricks-Ferguson VL, Pearson J, et al. Development of an in-home standardized end-of-life treatment program for pediatric patients dying of brain tumors. *J Spec Pediatr Nurs*. 2013; 18(2): 144–57.

25. American Academy of Pediatrics, Committee on Bioethics and Committee on Hospital Care. Palliative care for children. *Pediatrics*. 2000; 106(2): 351–7.

26. Pearn J. Incidence, prevalenceand gene frequency studies of chronic childhood spinal muscular atrophy. *J Med Genet*. 1978; 15(6): 409–13.

27. Battista V, Mosher P. Spinal muscular atrophy. In: Ferguson-Hendricks V., ed. *Palliative Care for Pediatric Life-Limiting Conditions*. Pittsburgh, PA: Hospice and Palliative Nurses Association; 2014:165–86.

28. Santucci G. Pain management for children with life-limiting conditions and at the end of life. In: Santucci G, ed. *Core Curriculum for the Pediatric Hospice and Palliative Nurse*. Pittsburgh, PA: Hospice and Palliative Nurses Association; 2011:43–66.

29. Crosta QR, Ward TM, Walker AJ, et al. A review of pain measures for hospitalized children with cognitive impairment. *J Spec Pediatr Nurs*. 2014; 19(2): 109–18.

30. Friedrichsdorf SJ, Kang TI. The management of pain in children with life-limiting illnesses. *Pediatr Clin North Am*. 2007; 54(5): 645–72.

31. McSherry M, Kehoe K, Carroll JM, et al. Psychosocial and spiritual needs of children living with a life-limiting illness. *Pediatr Clin North Am*. 2007; 54(5): 609–29.

32. Office of the Legislative Counsel, U.S. House of Representatives. Compilation of Patient Protection and Affordable Care Act, As Amended Through May 1, 2010, Including Patient Protection and Affordable Care Act Health-Related Portions of the Health Care and Education Reconciliation Act of 2010, Legislative Counsel, 111th Congress 2d Session, Print 111-1, 202–203.

Chapter 15

Palliative Care of the Geriatric Patient

Phyllis B. Whitehead

Key Point

- More than 50% of all deaths, most of whom are geriatric patients, occur in the acute care setting, where the focus is on active, curative treatment, not on managing symptoms and establishing realistic goals of care.

Introduction

Seriously ill, hospitalized patients represent a specialized patient population that greatly benefit from the expanded skills and knowledge of palliative APRNs. These patients and their loved ones have unique needs that are often unaddressed in a busy healthcare system. By the year 2030, almost one in five adults will be over the age of 65 years and have at least one chronic illness.[1–3] Often, chronically ill patients have uncertain prognoses and poorly predictable disease trajectories, resulting in numerous emergency department visits and hospital admissions.

Chronic Kidney Disease

See Table 15.1 for the stages of chronic kidney disease.

End-Stage Renal Disease

With the growing elderly population, the number of patients with acute kidney injury, stage 4 and 5 chronic kidney disease, or end-stage renal disease (ESRD) and comorbidities is increasing.[6–8] Mortality among ESRD patients is 10–100 times greater than in the general population when matched for age and gender.[7] The number of patients receiving dialysis is increasing by up to 10% annually, and the number of those older than 75 years undergoing dialysis has doubled over the past 20 years.[7] In 2000, the American Society of Nephrology and Renal Physicians Association published the first clinical practice guideline encouraging palliative care for ESRD patients. It was revised

Table 15.1 Stages of Chronic Kidney Disease		
Stage	Glomerular Filtration Rate (GFR)	Status
1	>90	Normal kidney function
2	60–89	Declining GFR with comorbidities
3	30–59	Decline, incidence of anemia, malnutrition, poor quality of life, consider palliative care consult
4	15–29	Pre-dialysis, preparation for dialysis
5	<15	Renal replacement therapy, kidney transplant, or hospice care

Adapted from references 4 and 5.

in 2010 to include information on an integrated prognostic model predicting the mortality of hemodialysis patients (available at http://touch-calc.com/calculators/sq).[8,9]

Patients, loved ones, and hospitals need to be prepared to have conversations about serious illness, advanced illness, and end of life, ideally before dialysis is initiated but most certainly when patients are functionally and physically declining despite dialysis. APRNs need to feel comfortable having the discussion with patients and their families regarding whether dialysis may offer a better quality and quantity of life compared to conservative management of symptoms.[7] For example, patients older than 80 years who start dialysis experience a significant loss of functionality within the first 6 months of treatment, requiring caregiver support or placement in a nursing home.[6] Unfortunately, randomized clinical trials evaluating the benefits of dialysis for older adults are lacking.[7,10]

Paramount is the collaboration with the hospital's nephrologists and the dialysis nurses to implement the American Society of Nephrology and Renal Physicians Association's published clinical practice guidelines for palliative care counseling and symptom management. Early palliative care involvement and integration into routine ESRD management are preferred for creating trusting relationships with patients and their loved ones. Several instruments have been developed by Cohen and colleagues—such as the Dialysis Discontinuation Quality of Dying (DDQOD) and the Dialysis Quality of Dying Apgar (QODA)—which help distinguish between good and bad deaths for dialysis patients and may assist with end-of-life discussions.[10,11]

Palliative care renal literature and guidelines suggest that the elements of good end-of-life care for ESRD patients include: advance care planning for agreed level of care and preferred place of care; appropriate transition from life-sustaining to comfort care, including potential withdrawal of dialysis; ongoing dialogues with patients and caregivers regarding prognosis and treatment options; and aggressive symptom management throughout disease progression.[8]

Physical assessment includes the presence of skin turgor and color changes (i.e., gray-bronze color); oliguria or anuria; edema and/or ascites; jugular vein distention; fluid accumulation in the lungs; blood pressure and orthostatic changes; fluid retention resulting in weight gain; hypocalcemia; dry, flaky skin; ammonia-smelling breath; tremors/seizures; easy bruising; and signs of anemia.[4] Routine laboratory tests should be ordered, including blood urea nitrogen (BUN), creatinine, hemoglobin, hematocrit, calcium, phosphorus, sodium, and potassium. Other diagnostic testing may involve imaging (computed tomography [CT] or magnetic resonance imaging [MRI]); renal arteriograms; and kidney, ureters, and bladder (KUB) radiographs.[4] The APRN should assess for common symptoms, such as nausea and vomiting, anxiety, depression, constipation, diarrhea, pruritus, pain, fatigue, and anorexia. Morphine should be avoided; fentanyl, methadone, and oxycodone are preferred in the treatment of pain.[4,12]

All reversible causes should be eliminated, especially in the treatment of acute renal failure. For ESRD, dialysis discussions should cover lifestyle changes, dietary restrictions, symptom management, potential complications, transplant options, and whether dialysis will continue until the patient dies or under what circumstances dialysis will be discontinued.[4,5] Once a decision is made to stop dialysis, all nonessential medications must be stopped to avoid toxicities and to stop or at least minimize fluid volume. Patient and family education must be provided on what to expect, especially alleviating the fear of "drowning in fluids" that accompanies stopping dialysis. The patient's diet should be liberalized so he or she can enjoy foods and beverages that have been restricted. The patient who stops dialysis has a prognosis usually measured in days to a few weeks. The APRN should review disposition planning options with the patient and family, including home with hospice, long-term care facility with hospice, or a residential hospice facility, and provide guidance in this decision.

Dementia

Dementia is a common diagnosis on medical, surgical, and geriatric units. Frequently, families do not understand that dementia is a life-limiting condition. APRNs are uniquely positioned to initiate conversations to help families understand the disease trajectory for dementia patients. The incidence of dementia is growing; it occurs in approximately 1% of all people 65 years of age and 50% of people aged 90 years.[13] Worldwide, 24 million individuals are living with dementia, and this number is predicted to double over the next 20 years.[13] Dementia, specifically Alzheimer's disease, is the fifth leading cause of death.[14] Dementia is a progressive, incurable condition that causes limitations in life and should be recognized as a life-limiting condition.[13,15–17]

Dementia can have many causes, such as Alzheimer's disease, vascular dementia, advanced Parkinson's or Huntington's disease, Lewy body disease, and excessive and chronic alcohol use.[17] Impairments in mental and physical functioning, such as memory loss, language impairment, personality changes, dysphagia, and inability to perform activities of daily living, characterize the condition.[13,17] There are seven stages of dementia (Table 15.2). The APRN should be familiar with these stages to help clinicians and families understand the role of palliative and hospice care for patients and their loved ones.

Table 15.2 Stages of Dementia	
Stage	Impairment Level
1	No impairment
2	Very mild decline—unnoticeable memory lapses
3	Mild decline—noticeable memory and concentration problems; losing items
4	Moderate decline—forgetfulness of events; difficulty performing tasks
5	Moderate to severe decline—gaps in memory, thinking; needs help with activities of daily living
6	Severe decline—loss of awareness of recent experiences; remembers own name but has difficulty with others
7	Very severe decline—total care; swallowing impaired; hospice eligible

Adapted from references 17 and 18.

Evidence shows that patients with end-stage dementia are less likely to be referred to palliative care than other non-oncological end-stage disease patients (9% vs. 25%), and dementia patients are likely to be prescribed fewer palliative medications (28% vs. 51%).[19] Caregivers' burden can be worsened when periods of stability are interrupted by acute exacerbations—in contrast to the more predictable decline in patients with advanced cancer.[19] Advance care planning and goal setting should be initiated early in the disease progression, while the patient can provide guidance to loved ones. Due to the progression of dementia, it can be challenging for family and clinicians to know when to initiate palliation as a goal.

The use of functionality and cognition scales, such as the Minimum Data Set 2 (MDS-2) or the Functional Assessment Staging (FAST) instruments, can be helpful in quantifying the stage and identifying appropriate palliative and/or hospice patients.[16,20] Both pain (39%) and dyspnea (46%) are common symptoms at end of life for many dementia patients,[18] and these conditions should be aggressively treated on a first-line basis with an opioid such as morphine. Patients with dementia receive less analgesia than patients who are cognitively intact. They often cannot express themselves verbally and hence receive suboptimal palliative care.[13] The APRN should integrate the use of behavioral pain assessment tools, such as the Pain Assessment in Advanced Dementia Scale (PAINAD). The American Society of Pain Management Nursing's *Position Statement on Pain Assessment in Patients Unable to Self-Report* recommends using patient self-report of pain if possible, review of known pain etiologies from the medical history, observation of pain-related behaviors, and family or proxy reports to assess for pain in the dementia patient.[18] Agitation may affect up to half of end-stage dementia patients, necessitating a calm environment and the treatment of reversible causes, such as pain, dyspnea, and constipation.[18,21] The APRN should assess for cognitive changes, including delirium. Tools such as the Mini-Mental State Examination (MMSE), the Short Portable Mental Status Questionnaire (SPMSQ), the Delirium Observation Screening Scale, and the Confusion Assessment Method (CAM) can be used to screen for cognitive changes and delirium to enhance symptom management.[18]

Infections, such as pneumonia from aspiration, urinary tract infections, or pressure ulcers from lack of mobility are a natural part of the disease progression.[18] The APRN must discuss with caregivers the role of antibiotics in the context of a life-prolonging intervention, especially in the late stages of the disease. Antibiotics are not benign and can cause complications such as *Clostridium difficile* infection, so an early dialogue is warranted about the use of oral and/or intravenous antibiotics as contingent on the patient's goals of care.[18,20]

Due to the prevalence of dysphagia (93%),[17] malnutrition and dehydration are common. Conversations on the use of artificial hydration and nutrition should start early and be revisited as the disease progresses. A speech-language pathologist referral should be considered to determine the safest oral intake/diet recommendations for the patient.

Frequently, loved ones ask how we can allow the patient to "starve to death." A candid discussion on the natural dying process for a dementia patient is imperative. Using a careful selection of words such as "fasting" and explaining that this process is not uncomfortable can be helpful for caregivers. Comparing the fasting state to a time when the loved one has been ill and did not have a desire to eat may also be helpful. It is important to emphasize that the patient will be offered comfort foods and/or sips of beverages, despite the risk of aspiration, along with frequent oral care. Providing the information and allowing loved ones time to process it while providing empathy are essential APRN skills.

Hip Fractures

Elderly patients hospitalized for hip fractures are common on medical-surgical units. In 2010, 258,000 hospital admissions were for hip fractures among patients aged 65 and older.[22] By 2030, hip fractures are projected to increase by 12.6% to 289,000 admissions.[22] Although one may not consider consulting palliative care for a hip fracture alone, it may be appropriate if the patient has multiple comorbidities (e.g., heart failure, dementia, chronic pulmonary and kidney disease) and is frail even at baseline. Hip fractures in a patient older than 65 years should trigger a palliative care consult.

Having a goals-of-care conversation with the patient and family can align the patient's priorities of care (cure vs. quality of life) while ensuring that both surgical and conservative intervention options are fully discussed, including the benefits and risks (mortality) of each. Many times, the patient's main priority is to ambulate again, so surgery may be the better option if, realistically, rehabilitation is possible. It is important for patients and their loved ones to understand that pain and symptom management can be achieved via medical management.

Hip fractures increase especially after the age of 60 and then exponentially after the age of 80.[22–24] Approximately 30% of community-dwelling senior citizens age 65 and older fall annually, with higher numbers in institutions.[24] Hip fractures are disabling and a major cause of morbidity and mortality in elderly individuals.[22] Common risk factors for falls include: cognitive dysfunction;

bowel/bladder incontinence; medications, such as opioids, sedatives, and diuretics; impaired balance; environmental hazards, such as throw rugs and slippery floors; pets; and weakness/instability.[18]

Chronic Obstructive Pulmonary Disease

Chronic obstructive pulmonary disease (COPD) is the third leading cause of death in the United States and is predicted to become the third leading cause of death worldwide by 2020.[5,25,26] The death rate due to COPD continues to rise.[27,28] COPD is commonly seen later in life after exposure to risk factors such as cigarette smoking, tuberculosis, and noxious gaseous/particulate matter, and a history of respiratory infections. COPD is progressive and incurable; it is punctuated by acute exacerbations characterized by airflow obstruction caused by chronic inflammation.[26]

The last years of life for COPD patients are tainted by progressive functional decline, poor quality of life, and oxygen dependency.[27,28] Death usually occurs from acute exacerbations of COPD, such as lung infections, respiratory failure, and secondary complications from comorbidities.[27] Hospital admissions increase with age, with patients older than 80 years at the highest risk of hospitalization (14 times greater than 40- to 49-year-old patients).[28]

Common symptoms are anxiety, cough, sputum production, dyspnea, and fever. The prevalence of dyspnea is 90–95% in COPD patients.[25] Physical

Table 15.3 Pharmacologic Management of COPD

Medication	Onset of Action	Mechanism of Action	Dosing Schedule
Albuterol	5–15 mins	SMR	Varies
Levalbuterol	5–10 mins	SMR	Varies
Ipratropium	<15 mins	SMR	Varies
Formoterol	<10 mins	SMR	Bid
Arformoterol	7–20 mins	SMR	Bid
Tiotropium	<30 mins	SMR	Daily
Budesonide	Varies	Anti-inflammatory	Bid/Tid
Fluticasone/salmeterol inhaler	2 hours	SMR/anti-inflammatory	Bid
Budesonide/formoterol inhalation	2 hours	SMR/anti-inflammatory	Bid
Aminophylline	Varies	SMR	Daily
Theophylline	Varies	SMR	Daily
Roflumilast	Up to 8 hours	Anti-inflammatory	Daily
Prednisone	1–2 hours	Anti-inflammatory	Daily
Methylprednisolone	1–2 hours	Anti-inflammatory	Daily
Fluticasone	Up to 2 weeks	Anti-inflammatory	Bid

SMR = Smooth Muscle Relaxant
Adapted from references 25 and 29.

assessment findings include audible wheezing; abnormal breath sounds (rhonchi, crackles; decreased breath sounds; paradoxical respirations; tachypnea and tachycardia; dyspnea; "blue bloater" (classic sign of bronchitis); "pink puffer" (sign of emphysema); accessory muscle use; fever; cough; cyanosis; dependent edema; weight loss; fatigue; sleep deprivation; changes in mental status; depression; and anxiety.[25]

Laboratory tests routinely ordered include chemistries to monitor elevated serum carbon dioxide levels and arterial blood gas analysis for acidosis, hypercapnia, and hypoxemia. Pulse oximetry may be helpful in detecting hypoxemia. Chest radiographs and chest (CT) imaging are useful in revealing fibrosis, effusions, hyperinflated lungs, and hyperlucent areas reflecting bullae.[25] Low-dose opioids are the first line for the treatment of dyspnea, whereas benzodiazepines are the first line for treating anxiety, and best practice suggests a low-dose opioid (which may be contrary to how clinicians

Table 15.4 COPD Grading per GOLD

Airflow Limitation	Post-bronchodilator Spirometry	Descriptors
GOLD 1 Mild	FEV_1 ≥80% of predicted normal values FEV_1/FVC <70% confirms COPD diagnosis.	• Mild airflow limitation • May be unaware that lung function has started to decline • May not have COPD symptoms • May have symptoms of chronic cough and excessive mucus • Rarely seek treatment
GOLD 2 Moderate	50 ≤ FEV_1 <80% predicted values	• Airflow limitation worsens. • May notice symptoms, particularly shortness of breath upon exertion • Cough and sputum production • Many people typically seek treatment at this stage.
GOLD 3 Severe	30 ≤ FEV_1 <50% predicted values	• Airflow significantly worsens. • Shortness of breath becomes more evident and COPD exacerbation is common. • Decrease in activity tolerance and increase in fatigability
GOLD 4 Very Severe	FEV_1 <30% of predicted normal values **or** FEV_1 <50% of predicted normal values plus chronic respiratory failure	• Quality of life is greatly impaired. • COPD exacerbations are life-threatening. • Airflow limitation is severe. • Chronic respiratory failure is often present at this stage and may lead to complications, such as cor pulmonale and/or, eventually, death. • Hospice eligible

FEV_1, forced expiratory volume in 1 second; FVC, forced vital capacity
Adapted from references 5 and 25.

have been trained).[25,29] Optimizing medication management of the underlying pulmonary disease is key to good palliative treatment of the COPD patient. Table 15.3 discusses pharmacologic management of COPD.

COPD is a common primary diagnosis for an acute care admission. Disease progression often includes frequent admissions and escalation of care, such as intensive care. Multiple admissions to the hospital for the same reason should trigger a palliative care consult. The disease trajectory is challenging, as is prognostication, because death frequently occurs before the patient is perceived as terminal.[26] COPD grading per the Global Initiative for COPD (GOLD)[5,25] is a helpful tool in prognostication (Table 15.4).

COPD patients and their families must understand their disease progression, future care, and end-of-life treatment options.[26]

Conclusion

With the majority of deaths occurring in acute care settings, care often includes active, curative treatment with less focus on symptom management or establishing realistic goals of care. Geriatric patients have many comorbidities such as kidney disease, dementia, and hip fractures that are best proactively managed. They may benefit from palliative care.

References

1. Garner KK, Goodwin JA, McSweeney JC, Kirchner JE. Nurse executives' perceptions of end-of-life care provided in hospitals. *J Pain Symptom Manage*. 2013; 45(2): 235–43.

2. Gott M, Ingleton C, Gardiner C, et al. How to improve end of life care in acute hospitals. *Nurs Older People*. 2009; 21(7): 26–9.

3. Reed SM. A unitary-caring conceptual model for advanced practice nursing in practice care. *Holist Nurs Pract*. 2010; 24(1): 23–34.

4. Gorman L. Renal conditions. In: Dahlin CM, Lynch MT, eds. *Core Curriculum for the Advanced Practice Hospice and Palliative Registered Nurse*. 2nd ed. Pittsburgh, PA: Hospice and Palliative Nurses Association; 2013: 353–68.

5. Maxwell TL. Caring for those with chronic illness. In: Ferrell B, Coyle N, eds. *Oxford Textbook of Palliative Nursing*. 3rd ed. New York, NY: Oxford University Press; 2010: 690–7.

6. Arulkumaran N, Szawarski P, Philips BJ. End-of-life care in patients with end-stage renal disease. *Nephrol Dial Transplant*. 2012; 27: 879–81.

7. Koshy AN, Mace R, Youl L, Challenor S, Bull R, Fassett RG. Contrasting approaches to end of life and palliative care in end kidney disease. *Indian J Nephrol*. 2012; 22(4): 307–9.

8. McAdoo SP, Brown EA, Chesser AM, Farrington K, Salisbury EM. Measuring the quality of end of life management in patients with advanced kidney disease: results from the Pan-Thames Renal Audit Group. *Nephrol Dial Transplant*. 2011; 27: 1548–54.

9. Moss AH. Revised dialysis clinical practice guideline promotes more informed decision-making. *Clin J Am Soc Nephrol*. 2010; 5: 2380–3.

10. Mid-Atlantic Renal Coalition and the Kidney End-of-Life Coalition. *Clinical algorithm & preferred medications to treat pain in dialysis patients.* MidAtlantic Renal Coalition and the Kidney End-of-Life Coalition. Available at http://www.kidneysupportivecare.org/Files/PainBrochure9-09.aspx. Published March 13, 2009. Accessed October 23, 2016.

11. Renal Physicians Association. *Shared Decision-Making in the Appropriate Initiation and Withdrawal from Dialysis. Clinical Practice Guideline.* 2nd ed. Available at file:///C:/Users/connied/Downloads/Shared%20Decision%20Making%20Toolkit%20(1).pdf. Published September 25, 2010. Accessed October 23, 2016.

12. Quill TE, Bower KA, Holloway RG, et al. Pain management. In: *Primer of Palliative Care.* 6th ed. Chicago, IL: American Academy of Hospice and Palliative Medicine; 2014:17.

13. Brorson H, Plymoth R, Ormon K, Bolmsjo I. Pain relief at the end of life: nurses' experiences regarding end-of-life pain relief in patients with dementia. *Pain Management Nursing.* 2014; 15(1): 315–23.

14. Smith LW, Amell E, Edlund B, Mueller M. A dimensional analysis of the concept of suffering in people with dementia at end of life. *J Hospice Palliative Nurs.* 2014; 16(5): 263–70.

15. Boogaard JA, van Soest-Poortvliet MC, Anema JR, et al. Feedback on end-of-life care in dementia: the study protocol of the follow-up project. *BMC Palliative Care.* 2013; 12(29): 1–8.

16. Coleman AME. End-of-life issues in caring for patients with dementia: the case for palliative care in management of terminal dementia. *Am J Hospice Palliative Med.* 2012; 29(1): 9–12.

17. Dahlin CM, Cohen AK, Goldsmith T. Dysphagia, xerostomia, and hiccups. In: Ferrell B, Coyle N, eds. *Oxford Textbook of Palliative Nursing.* 4th ed., New York, NY: Oxford University Press; 2015:191–216.

18. Smeltz R. Neurological conditions. In: Dahlin CM, Lynch MT, eds. *Core Curriculum for the Advanced Practice Hospice and Palliative Registered Nurse.* 2nd ed. Pittsburgh, PA: Hospice and Palliative Nurses Association; 2013:389–418.

19. Costa-Requena G, Espinosa Val M, Cristofol R. Caregiver burden in end-of-life care: advanced cancer and final stage of dementia. *Palliat Support Care.* 2014: 13(3): 1–7.

20. Parsons C, McCorry N, Murphy K, et al. Assessment of factors that influence physician decision making regarding medication use in patients with dementia at the end of life. *Int J Geriatric Psychiatry.* 2014; 29: 281–90.

21. Quill TE, Bower KA, Holloway RG, Shah MS, Caprio TV, Storey CP. Delirium, depression and anxiety, and fatigue. In: *Primer of Palliative Care.* 6th ed. Chicago, IL: American Academy of Hospice and Palliative Medicine; 2014:91–111.

22. Yoon B, Baek J, Kim MK, Lee Y, Ha Y, Koo K. Poor prognosis in elderly patients who refused surgery because of economic burden and medical problem after hip fracture. *J Korean Med Sci.* 2013; 28: 1378–81.

23. Alarcon T, Gonzalez-Montalvo JI, Gotor P, Madero R, Otero A. A new hierarchical classification for prognosis of hip fracture after 2 years' follow up. *J Nutr Health Aging.* 2010; 15(10): 919–23.

24. Kristensen MT. Factors affecting functional prognosis of patients with hip fracture. *Eur J Physical Rehab Med.* 2011; 47(2): 257–64.

25. Bouxman SR. Pulmonary conditions. In: Dahlin CM, Lynch MT, eds. *Core Curriculum for the Advanced Practice Hospice and Palliative Registered Nurse.* 2nd ed. Pittsburgh, PA: Hospice and Palliative Nurses Association; 2013:331–51.

26. Momen N, Hadfield P, Kuhn I, Smith E, Barclay S. Discussing an uncertain future: end-of-life care conversations, in chronic obstructive pulmonary disease. A systematic literature review and narrative synthesis. *Thorax.* 2012; 67: 777–80.

27. Chou W, Lai Y, Huang Y, Chang C, Wu W, Hung Y. Comparing end-of-life care for hospitalized patients with chronic obstructive pulmonary disease and lung cancer in Taiwan. *J Palliative Care.* 2013; 29(1): 29–35.

28. Chou W, Lai Y, Hung Y. Comparing end-of-life care in hospitalized patients with chronic obstructive pulmonary disease with and without palliative care in Taiwan. *J Research Med Sci.* 2013; 18(7): 594–600.

29. Quill TE, Bower KA, Holloway RG, et al. Dyspnea. In: *Primer of Palliative Care.* 6th ed. Chicago, IL: American Academy of Hospice and Palliative Medicine; 2014:50–51.

Index

References to tables, figures, and boxes are indicated by italicized *t*, *f*, and *b*

CPSIA information can be obtained
at www.ICGtesting.com
Printed in the USA
BVHW070726010323
659314BV00004B/12